Manual of Health Assessment

Manual of Health Assessment

Helen Nelson Carcio, R.N., C., M.S.
Assistant Professor, Curry College, Milton, MA

Little, Brown and Company
Boston   Toronto

Library of Congress Cataloging in Publication Data

Carcio, Helen Nelson.
  Manual of health assessment.

  Includes index.
  1. Nursing—Handbooks, manuals, etc. 2. Diagnosis—
Handbooks, manuals, etc. I. Title. [DNLM: 1. Holistic
Health. 2. Medical History Taking—nurses' instruction.
3. Nursing Process. 4. Physical Examination—methods—
nurses' instruction. WY 100 C265m]
RT48.C36   1985   616.07′5   85-4732
ISBN 0-316-12850-3

Library of Congress Catalog Card No. 85–4732

ISBN 0-316-12850-3

9 8 7 6 5 4 3 2

HAL

Published simultaneously in Canada
by Little, Brown & Company (Canada) Limited

Printed in the United States of America

Illustrator: Bernadette L. Hunter, Newmarket, Ontario

Credits

Figs. 1–2, 2–3, 6–8, 9–9, 9–11: Josephine M. Sana and
Richard D. Judge (Eds.), *Physical Assessment Skills for
Nursing Practice* (2nd ed.), Boston: Little, Brown, 1982.
Figs. 2–1, 6–12, 9–2, 10–4, 10–5, 12–4, 13–4, 13–6, 13–8,
13–10, 13–13, 13–16, 13–20, 13–22, 13–23, 13–24, and
Tabs. 14–1, 14–3: Richard D. Judge, George D. Zuidema,
and Faith T. Fitzgerald, *Clinical Diagnosis: A Physiologic
Approach* (4th ed.), Boston: Little, Brown, 1982.
Figs. 7–2, 11–2: William H. Masters, Virginia E. Johnson,
and Robert C. Kolodny, *Human Sexuality* (2nd ed.),
Boston: Little, Brown, 1985.
Fig. 9–14: Richard S. Snell, *Clinical Anatomy for Medical
Students* (2nd ed.), Boston: Little, Brown, 1981.
Figs. 12–8, 12–9: Thomas H. Green, Jr., *Gynecology:
Essentials of Clinical Practice* (3rd ed.), Boston: Little,
Brown, 1977.
Fig. 14–11: John F. Simpson and Kenneth R. Magee,
Clinical Evaluation of the Nervous System, Boston: Little,
Brown, 1973.

To my husband Frank,
my three sons, Marc, Benjamin, and Christian John,
and to my parents Helen and Nels Nelson,
with love and affection.

Contents

Preface

The purpose of this manual is to provide a holistic and systematic approach to health assessment. The logical sequence of the examination as described provides the examiner with a framework for effective decision making in the application of the nursing process.

The book begins with an introduction outlining the comprehensive health history. The chapters that follow are organized by major body regions, with emphasis on the young to middle-aged adult. Differences in the implications for the assessment process or findings for the child, the adolescent, and the geriatric client are integrated throughout.

The chapters are unique in their format. The right hand pages of the manual contain information directly related to the health assessment process. The left hand pages contain related facts intended to clarify the information on the right. They are comprised of definitions, helpful hints, illustrations, photographs, and tables. Any word defined on a left page is in boldfaced italic type on the facing page to alert the examiner to the presence of the definition. The helpful hints relate to the examination techniques, and are integrated into the discussion of the examination by the use of a degree symbol (°). The diagrams, illustrations, and photographs are referenced by a figure number, directing the examiner to the left side of the manual.

Chapters are organized according to the same structure: each begins with specific clinical considerations necessary for assessment. These provide the examiner with pertinent information and strategies that increase the effectiveness of the examination. A format for relevant history questions to ask the client follows. The specific questions are listed on the right hand page, while the explanation of their relevance is explained on the facing page.

The next chapter section presents the basic techniques of inspection, palpation, percussion, and auscultation as related to the specific body system being discussed. Within each technique, the health assessment of the client proceeds in a logical sequence:

Equipment—an identification of any equipment to be used.

Position—a description of the position the client should assume for a particular maneuver.

Instructions to the client—a unique section incorporating the principles of patient teaching, and including information about what the client should expect during that portion of the examination as well as an explanation of any maneuvers that he or she might be asked to perform.

Technique—a step-by-step outline of how the examiner should carry out the actual technical aspect of the physical examination.

Note—a list of possible signs that may indicate disease to be used as a point of reference, for correlating findings actually noted during the examination.

Normal findings—findings regarded as typical or usual in a healthy individual.

Clinical alterations—a list of common alterations and the disease(s) they are commonly associated with. These are examples of possible systemic manifestations and are not intended to be a detailed description of a specific disease process.

Each chapter concludes with a sample recording of what to chart for a normal client.

The preparation of *Manual of Health Assessment* was exciting and challenging. It was only made possible through the love, support, and guidance of many people.

Special thanks:

To my three sisters—Anita Britton for her modeling, Bernadette Hunter for her creative illustrations, M. Christine Nelson for her photographs and musculoskeletal illustrations;

To other family members who served as models—Kelly Britton, Christian Carcio, Ben Carcio, Marc Carcio, Mary Hunter, and Helen Nelson;

To the following physicians who contributed their medical expertise and personal support: David Cochran, Braintree, MA; Michael Drew, Boston, MA; Charles Gaughan, South Weymouth, MA; Donald Peter Goldstein, Boston, MA; Andrew Merliss, South Weymouth, MA; John R. Saunders, Jr., Towson, Maryland; and to L. L. Eldredge, Hingham, MA, who kept my children well enough to give me the time to complete this manual;

To my friends and colleagues who contributed their guidance and support: Carol Barrett, Linda Jarvis, Elizabeth Kudzma, Lou Levin, Gretchen Mayher, Carol Robinson, Robbie Robinson, Ann Roy, Sarah Wriston, the graduate students and faculty in Primary Care at Simmons College, Boston, MA, and the nursing students and administration and faculty of Curry College, Milton, MA;

To the faith of Julie Stillman, Nursing editor, Little, Brown and Company, to the enthusiastic support and encouragement of Ann West, Editor, College Division, Little, Brown and Company, and to Lauren Green, Book Editor, Little, Brown and Company, for putting it all together;

To Sue McCarthy for her support, editorial advice, and manuscript preparation; and to Bruce Pestilli, photographer, for his technical assistance.

Helen Nelson Carcio

Contributing Authors

Susan E. Blankenship, R.N., C., M.S.
Assistant Professor and Clinical Coordinator
Graduate Program in Primary Health Care Nursing
Simmons College
Boston, Massachusetts;
Adult Nurse Practitioner
Brigham and Womens Hospital
Boston, Massachusetts

Ann H. Gough, R.N., M. Ed., C.N.R.N.
Instructor of Nursing
New England Deaconess Hospital School of Nursing
Boston, Massachusetts

Dennis Hines, R.N., M.S.N., C.F.N.P.
Occupational Health Service
Sturdy Memorial Hospital
Attleboro, Massachusetts

Martha Kleinerman Tabas, R.N., C., M.S.
Gynecology Nurse Practitioner
Crittenton-Hastings House Clinic
Brighton, Massachusetts;
Former Assistant Professor
Primary Health Care Nursing
Simmons College
Boston, Massachusetts

Patricia J. Shelman, R.N., M.A.
Oncology Nurse Specialist
Framingham Union Hospital
Framingham, Massachusetts

Manual of Health Assessment

General Principles of Health Assessment

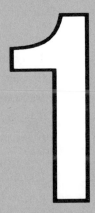

Health assessment is an integral part of the assessment portion of the nursing process. It includes the skillful collection of subjective data during the interview; the analysis of objective data obtained by inspection, palpation, percussion, and auscultation of each body system; and the synthesis of the combined information to formulate a diagnosis. Proficiency in health assessment increases the practitioner's ability to make effective decisions in planning, implementing, and evaluating health care.

Obtaining an accurate health history is essential: pertinent information from the past is correlated to the actual or potential health problems of the client. The health history is a holistic approach to the assessment of persons as they adapt to past and present alterations in mental and physical well-being.

Communication skills are basic to the knowledge of every student and practitioner of nursing and therefore are not repeated in this manual. A brief summary of the components of the health history is presented. Specific questions are appropriately included in subsequent chapters with the assessment of each body system. If time or the client's condition is a factor, these relevant questions need only be addressed. Further history can be assessed at a more appropriate time.

Before conducting the interview to collect data, the atmosphere should be relaxed, with the client dressed and seated comfortably. The examiner should explain that he or she will be writing down some information as the interview progresses. Initially, using index cards may help guide the examiner through the complex collection of data so important sections are not overlooked. The examiner must also not miss a prime opportunity to include health teaching as various preventive measures are addressed during the review of systems. The format of the health history has a built-in system of checks and balances for the accurate collection of data.

The parts of the health history follow a standardized sequence. The components of the database are outlined as follows:

1. Biographic data

2. Source of referral

3. Chief complaint (CC): client's own description of the primary reason for his or her seeking health care; in quotations, and usually limited to three or four words

4. History of present illness (HPI): chronologically covers all events from the onset of the illness to the health interview, and is organized in a logical sequence

    a. Dates of initial onset and subsequent episodes

    b. Setting

    c. Duration

    d. Timing

    e. Characteristic pattern

    f. Chronology

    g. Factors that aggravate the present illness

    h. Factors that relieve the present illness

    i. Associated signs and symptoms

    j. Psychological reaction to the illness

5. Prior medical history (PMH)

    a. General state of health

    b. Immunizations: type and date

    c. Childhood illnesses: nature and date

    d. Allergies: agent and reaction

    e. Hospitalizations, operations, or both: date, hospital, and reason

    f. Obstetric history

    g. History of blood transfusions

    h. Psychiatric history

    i. Current medications: ask particularly about over-the-counter drugs that the client may not view as medication

    j. Diet: 24-hour recall

    k. Sleep/rest pattern

    l. Habits: use of alcohol, tobacco, coffee, tea, or drugs

    m. Typical day

6. Family history: use a genogram (Fig. 1-1) to illustrate age and state of health, or age and cause of death, of grandparents, parents, siblings, spouses, and children; specifically address cancer, diabetes, hypertension, heart disease, kidney disease, arthritis, alcoholism, mental illness, and epilepsy (summarize as follows: family history negative for . . .; family history positive for . . .)

7. Psychosocial history: in paragraph form, include the following:

    a. Birthplace

    b. Educational level

    c. Military service

    d. Financial status

    e. Geographic exposure

    f. Life-style

    g. Hobbies and interests

    h. Outlook for the future

    i. Role relationship data

    j. Stress-management data

    k. Cognitive/perceptual data

8. Health maintenance to increase self-care

    a. Name of health-care provider

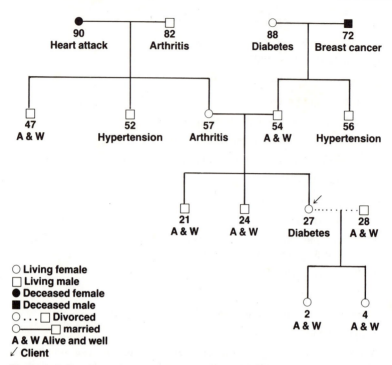

Figure 1–1. Sample genogram including parents, aunts, uncles, siblings, spouses, and children. Age of siblings increases from left to right.

   b. Exercise pattern

   c. Diet plan

   d. Special preventive health practices

   e. Mental health

9. Environmental assessment: past and present

   a. Home

   b. Employment

   c. Community

   d. Culture

10. Review of systems (ROS): an orderly review of subjective symptoms in each physiologic system; chart pertinent negatives and treat any positives as a chief complaint

   a. General: recent weight change, fatigue, fever

   b. Skin: recent change in texture of mole, dryness, rashes, pruritus, acne

   c. Hair: recent change in texture, alopecia, use of dyes

d. Nails: recent change in color or texture, nail-biting

e. Head: headache or injury

f. Eyes: injury, infections, pain, diplopia, blurring, excessive tearing, glaucoma, cataracts, photophobia, use of glasses or contact lenses, date of last eye examination

g. Ears: infection, loss of hearing, pain, discharge, tinnitis

h. Nose, nasopharynx, and sinuses: infections, pain, discharge, congestion, allergies, recent change in sense of smell

i. Mouth and throat: sore on lips or in mouth, bleeding and swollen gums, sore throat, history of streptococcal infections, difficulty swallowing, hoarseness, toothache, caries, date of last visit to dentist

j. Neck: swollen glands, goiter, pain, stiffness

k. Cardiovascular system: chest pain, palpitations, syncope, rheumatic fever, hypertension, varicosities, phlebitis, edema, results of past electrocardiogram or other cardiac tests

l. Respiratory system: cough, sputum production, chronic obstructive pulmonary disease (COPD), emphysema, shortness of breath, orthopnea (number of pillows the client uses at night), nocturnal dyspnea, chest pain, wheezing, hemoptysis, frequent upper respiratory tract infections, exposure to tuberculosis, date and results of last chest x-ray and tuberculosis test

m. Breast: self-examination, lesions, lumps, skin changes, nipple discharge, history of lumpectomy or mastectomy

n. Gastrointestinal system: nausea, vomiting, indigestion, heartburn, diarrhea, constipation, hemorrhoids, flatus, change in appetite or bowel pattern, color and consistency of stool

o. Genitourinary system: frequency, urgency, hesitency, nocturia, hematuria, incontinence, burning on urination, stones, excessive urination

p. Reproductive system, male: perineal rashes, testicular pain or masses, self-examination, lesions on genitals, use of birth control, infertility, history of venereal disease

q. Reproductive system, female: perineal rashes, lesions on genitals, use of birth control, menstrual history, obstetric history, infertility, use of tampons, history of venereal disease

r. Sexuality: orientation, frequency, satisfaction

s. Musculoskeletal system: muscular pain or cramps, injury, limitation of movement, pain or swelling of joints, backache

t. Neurologic system: paralysis, numbness, tingling, tremors, seizures, dizziness, fainting, loss of consciousness, memory changes

u. Psychiatric: anxiety, depression

v. Endocrine system: diabetes, thyroid disease

w. Hematologic system: anemia, easy bleeding, history of transfusions

The health history should be recorded in a brief outline and should be legible, neat, properly organized and clearly labeled. Underline the various section headings to provide further clarity and emphasis. Avoid excessive use of abbreviations. If information is not recorded accurately and completely, it does not matter how good the examiner's assessment technique is.

It is important for the examiner to understand the four basic techniques that are used when performing a physical examination. They are inspection, palpation, percussion, and auscultation. Health assessment of the client must be organized within the framework of these four techniques. Inspection is always performed first, followed by palpation (when examining tender areas, palpation is performed last). Findings are next confirmed through percussion and auscultation. Inspection and palpation may be used alone. Percussion and auscultation are particularly important when assessing the heart, lungs, abdomen, and joints.

The proper use of these techniques depends on the ability of the examiner to detect any deviation from normal and to assess its significance. The findings from the use of these techniques, in addition to the health history, increase the data base that enables the examiner to make accurate clinical judgments, concluding with a diagnosis.

In the following chapters, the techniques of inspection, palpation, percussion, and auscultation are described with applications to the examination of each body system.

Inspection is the critical observation of the client for any physical signs that indicate alteration from normal. It entails the visualization of an area noting its general appearance and any specific characteristics and the recognition of any disease components.

Inspection is the simplest technique to apply; unfortunately, it is the technique most often neglected. The examiner must remember to "look before touching." It is the technique of inspection that is always performed first and on which the other techniques are based. Inspection begins when the client enters the room, as the examiner generally assesses the physical characteristics of the client. These include gender, race, apparent age, general health state, nutritional status, grooming, motor activity, posture, and any appearance of disease. Additionally, inspection includes the assessment of mental status, noting mood, affect, expression, and mannerisms.

Color, size, location, texture, and contour of any abnormality; movement of affected limbs; and symmetry of the body should be visualized. Often contralateral sides of the body should be compared. Inspection also includes auditory and olfactory indicators (Fig. 1–2).

The room should be well lighted and warm. Draping should adequately expose the area to be examined.

Once these clues have been adequately assessed, the examiner proceeds to palpation, the sensitive assessment of feeling through touch. The examiner uses tactile, temperature, position, and vibratory senses. Accessible body parts are palpated to detect tenderness, texture, temperature, thrusts, thrills, crepitus, masses, vibrations, pulsations, contour, and mobility.

The examiner's hands should be warm and the area to be palpated should be fully exposed (Fig. 1–3). If anomalies are suspected by the client, the examiner should first assess the body part contralateral to the area of concern.

It is best to begin with light palpation and progress to deep palpation, palpating tender areas last. Prolonged pressure against the fingertips may dull

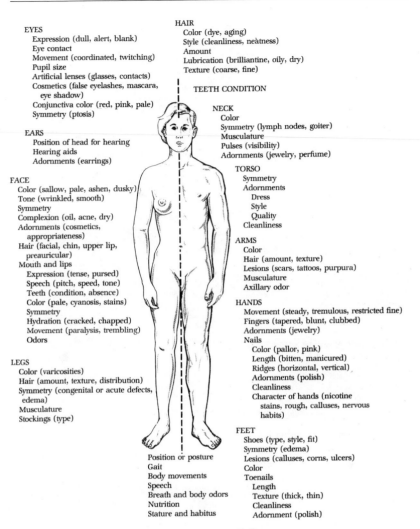

EYES
  Expression (dull, alert, blank)
  Eye contact
  Movement (coordinated, twitching)
  Pupil size
  Artificial lenses (glasses, contacts)
  Cosmetics (false eyelashes, mascara,
    eye shadow)
  Conjunctiva color (red, pink, pale)
  Symmetry (ptosis)

EARS
  Position of head for hearing
  Hearing aids
  Adornments (earrings)

FACE
  Color (sallow, pale, ashen, dusky)
  Tone (wrinkled, smooth)
  Symmetry
  Complexion (oil, acne, dry)
  Adornments (cosmetics,
    appropriateness)
  Hair (facial, chin, upper lip,
    preauricular)
  Mouth and lips
    Expression (tense, pursed)
    Speech (pitch, speed, tone)
    Teeth (condition, absence)
    Color (pale, cyanosis, stains)
    Symmetry
    Hydration (cracked, chapped)
    Movement (paralysis, trembling)
    Odors

LEGS
  Color (varicosities)
  Hair (amount, texture, distribution)
  Symmetry (congenital or acute defects,
    edema)
  Musculature
  Stockings (type)

HAIR
  Color (dye, aging)
  Style (cleanliness, neatness)
  Amount
  Lubrication (brilliantine, oily, dry)
  Texture (coarse, fine)

TEETH CONDITION

NECK
  Color
  Symmetry (lymph nodes, goiter)
  Musculature
  Pulses (visibility)
  Adornments (jewelry, perfume)

TORSO
  Symmetry
  Adornments
    Dress
    Style
    Quality
    Cleanliness

ARMS
  Color
  Hair (amount, texture)
  Lesions (scars, tattoos, purpura)
  Musculature
  Axillary odor

HANDS
  Movement (steady, tremulous, restricted fine)
  Fingers (tapered, blunt, clubbed)
  Adornments (jewelry)
  Nails
    Color (pallor, pink)
    Length (bitten, manicured)
    Ridges (horizontal, vertical)
    Adornments (polish)
    Cleanliness
    Character of hands (nicotine
      stains, rough, calluses, nervous
      habits)

FEET
  Shoes (type, style, fit)
  Symmetry (edema)
  Lesions (calluses, corns, ulcers)
  Color
  Toenails
    Length
    Texture (thick, thin)
    Cleanliness
    Adornment (polish)

Position or posture
Gait
Body movements
Speech
Breath and body odors
Nutrition
Stature and habitus

Figure 1–2. Physical appearance assessment guidelines.

tactile sensitivity. Palpation is slow and systematic. The examiner must always observe the client for any signs of discomfort.

Light palpation assesses superficial organs, pulsations, and muscle rigidity, and it often helps to relax the client, preparing him or her for the more uncomfortable deep palpation. Deep palpation is used to assess organs deep in the abdomen. When using the bimanual technique, the lower hand acts as the sensor, while the upper hand applies the pressure.

The tips of the fingers, or fingerpads, are most sensitive to discriminate texture and size, using the fingers for grasping. The dorsum of the hand is most

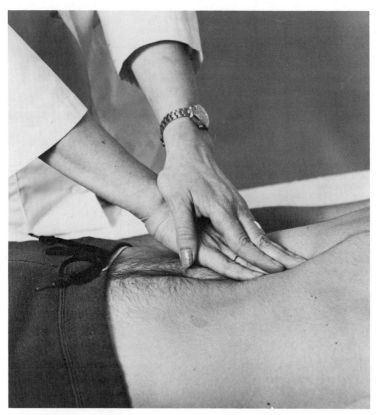

Figure 1–3. Bimanual palpation of the liver.

sensitive to any changes in body temperature. The palm, in the area of the metacarpal joints, is most sensitive to vibration (fremitus).

Percussion is the deliberate striking or tapping of a body part to elicit vibrations. The character of these vibrations assists the examiner in noting size, density, and location of an underlying structure. Sounds vary according to the degree of vibrations produced. Tissue or organs vibrate in inverse proportion to their density. The less dense an organ, the more it vibrates; the more dense, the less it vibrates. Percussion produces sounds of flatness, dullness, resonance, hyperresonance, and tympany.

The examiner must be familiar with the characteristics of these various sounds. These characteristics do not easily lend themselves to definition. Acquaintance with these sounds is best achieved by practicing on a healthy adult, or even on oneself. A flat sound can be elicited by striking a large muscle, such as the thigh. Dullness is best noted over an organ, such as the liver (seventh interspace on the right). Striking the intercostal spaces over the lungs produces

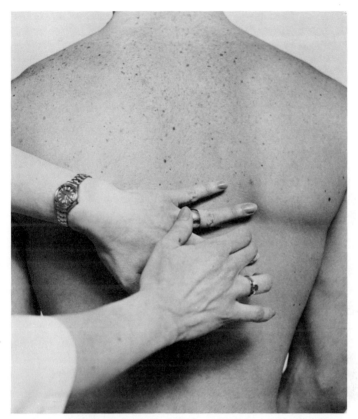

Figure 1–4. Percussion of the thorax. Note pleximeter is held parallel to client's ribs in the intercostal spaces.

resonance; over the bowel, tympany. Hyperresonance normally is not found on the healthy adult.

There are two types of percussion, mediate (indirect) and immediate (direct). Mediate percussion is the placement of a pleximeter—the middle or index finger—against the body area to be percussed. The tip of the middle finger (plexor) of the dominant hand strikes or taps the base of the distal phalanx of the pleximeter finger. The striking motion should come from the wrist, using a "flick of the wrist." The elbow and shoulder should remain stationary. The striking finger should be quickly removed to avoid dampening the transmitted sound. Also, the fingers and palm of the pleximeter hand should not rest on the body surface as they too may diminish the vibrations. The lightest percussion possible should be used to produce the desired effect.

Immediate percussion is performed by striking the body directly with the fingers or fist. It is particularly useful when eliciting tenderness over the kidneys or liver.

When performing percussion the examiner must note the pitch, duration,

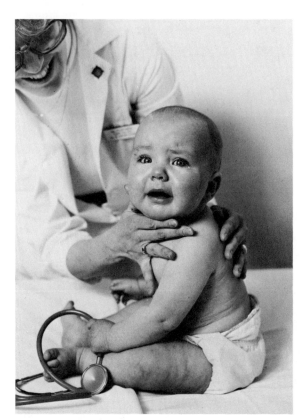

Figure 1–5. Allow a child to play with the stethoscope before attempting to auscultate the heart and lungs.

quality, and intensity of the various sounds. Two to three taps in each area is all that is necessary to assess these characteristics. Percussion is performed systematically, often comparing percussion notes on symmetric body parts.

Percussion is used primarily on the chest and abdomen. When percussing the lungs, the pleximeter finger should be placed parallel to the ribs, in the intercostal spaces (Fig. 1–4). Any change in percussion note is best assessed when percussing from areas of resonance to dull.

The examining room should be quiet. The examiner's hands should be warm and with nails trimmed. A child should be allowed to play with the stethoscope in order to decrease any fear of it (Fig. 1–5).

Organizing the findings assessed through inspection, palpation, and percussion, the examiner next proceeds to auscultation. Auscultation is the perception and interpretation of sound, most often through the use of a stethoscope. It is the technique most difficult to master for the beginning practitioner.

The ear must be trained to accurately recognize normal sounds and the specific characteristics of any abnormal sounds. The examiner must develop the ability to concentrate on one sound at a time and to note its relationship to other sounds auscultated. The examiner must note any variation in sound according to intensity (loudness), frequency (pitch), quality, and duration. Auscultation assesses crepitus in joints, vascular sounds such as bruits or murmurs, characteristics of breath and heart sounds, and the presence of bowel sounds.

Auscultation is performed systematically, often comparing symmetric body areas. The stethoscope should be warm and the room quiet. Any unnecessary movement of the stethoscope or breathing on the tubing should be avoided to eliminate any artifact. The diaphragm of the stethoscope assesses high-pitched sounds and should be held firmly against the client's body. The bell is used to detect low-pitched sounds and should be held lightly on the client's body.

Assessment of the Skin and Nails

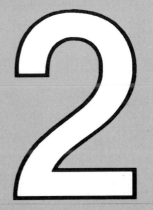

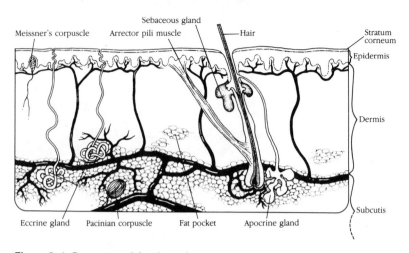

Figure 2–1. Structures of the skin.

Pruritus (itching). An unpleasant sensation carried by unmyelinated pain fibers, which a person attempts to relieve by scratching. It is the most common presenting symptom in skin disorders. It may be a symptom of either a primary skin disease or a serious disease of internal origin. The most common cause of generalized pruritus is excessive dryness of the skin, particularly in the elderly. Other conditions may be dermatologically, environmentally, systemically, or psychologically induced. If no lesion is apparent, systemic causes should be explored.

I. Clinical considerations

A. A thorough knowledge of the anatomy of the skin is essential (Fig. 2–1).

B. The examination of the skin includes inspection and palpation. The skin is readily accessible to both techniques.

C. The client may be asked to disrobe entirely for a general inspection, or the skin may be inspected as each area of the body is exposed during the physical examination.

D. Alterations in the color of the skin may be difficult to assess in persons with increased melanin. Areas where the skin's color can be assessed are the sclera, conjunctiva, mouth, palms, and soles.

E. The assessment of the skin yields valuable information to aid in identifying specific disorders or the presence of systemic disease.

F. Most descriptions of skin lesions refer to Caucasians; specific characteristics may vary with other races.

G. Good lighting, either natural or artificial, is essential when examining the skin and nails.

H. Pain sensation is often decreased in the elderly; pruritus is the predominant complaint.

II. Relevant history questions

A. *Pruritus,* **rashes, and lesions.** Ask questions related to the following:

    1. Onset, locations, pattern, spread, duration, distribution, characteristics of specific lesions, and history of previous episodes or allergies.

    2. Predisposing factors such as change in detergent or diet, sun exposure, season of the year, known exposure to an irritant, stress, or use of new medication.

    3. Associated signs and symptoms such as nausea, pain, jaundice, dryness of the skin, increased thirst, burning or tingling sensations.

    4. Use of therapeutic modalities.

B. **Change in color or texture of skin or nails.** Ask questions related to the following:

    1. Onset, location, pattern, spread, duration, and history of previous episodes.

    2. Predisposing factors such as exposure to local irritants or sun, topical applications, or stress.

    3. Associated signs and symptoms such as edema, shortness of breath, pruritus, or pain.

The functions of the skin include protection, regulation of body temperature, support of peripheral nerve endings, evaporation, production of vitamin D, and excretion.

Configuration and distribution of involved skin areas can best be assessed when standing away from the client.

The skin color is best assessed by examining areas that are not exposed to the sun. Color varies with sun and weather exposure and race.

Melanism. Increased production of melanin. Melanin is a major factor that determines the color of the skin.

Jaundice is accentuated in the forehead, nasolabial folds, palms, and soles.

Pallor is best assessed in the face, conjunctiva, and nails. It changes in response to the amount of oxygenated blood flowing to the skin surface.

Carotenemia. Deposits of carotene owing to excessive ingestion of pigmented vegetables. Carotene is found in oranges, carrots, apricots, and green vegetables. It does not stain the sclera as jaundice does.

Vitiligo. An acquired absence of melanocytes causing areas of hypopigmentation.

The oral mucosa does not contain keratin. It is pink because it is rich in oxygenated blood.

The mucous membrane is pigmented with melanin; the amount varies with race.

III. Inspection of the skin.° Position the client so that he or she is seated comfortably and draped appropriately with involved skin area exposed. Begin inspection 3 feet from the client to assess general skin condition or distribution and configuration of any lesions.° Then, closely inspect the characteristics of any lesions. A magnifying glass may be useful.

  A. Assess the color of the skin.°

    1. Note location, distribution, and appearance of any discolorations.

    2. Normal findings. Pinkish white to dark brown skin. Lighter pigmentation is present on the palms and soles of dark-skinned persons.

    3. Clinical alterations

        a. *Melanism* from scleredema, Addison's disease, or pernicious anemia.

        b. Cyanosis often from decreased oxygenation of the blood.

        c. Jaundice often from liver disease.°

        d. Pallor from decreased flow of oxyhemoglobin to the skin.°

        e. Erythema from fever, inflammation, infection, or burns.

        f. *Carotenemia* from increased ingestion of carotene.

        g. Bronze hues often from hemochromatosis in disorders of iron metabolism.

        h. *Vitiligo:* associated with albinism.

  B. Inspect the oral mucous membranes for color.

    1. Position. Client seated with mouth open.

    2. Note distribution and color of any discoloration.°

    3. Normal findings. Pale coral pink with varying amounts of melanin.°

    4. Clinical alterations

        a. Bright red from inflammation.

        b. Pallor from anemia or ischemia.

        c. Cyanosis from hypoxemia.

  C. Locate and describe any skin lesions or skin disorders.

    1. Technique. Diascopy: press microscope slide over lesion to accentuate its characteristics and to blanche surrounding area.

    2. Note

        a. Size and shape.

        b. Condition of surrounding skin.

        c. Distribution.

Annulur. Lesions arranged in circles.

Arciform. Lesions arranged in arcs.

Serpiginous. Lesions arranged in wavy lines.

Iris grouping. Lesions arranged in a bull's-eye shape.

Irregular. Lesions without a particular arrangement or pattern.

Zosteriform. Lesions arranged in broad bands occurring in areas supplied by the peripheral nerve roots.

Linear. Lesions along a straight line.

Keratosis. Superficial, benign, seborrheic warts that usually occur after the third decade.

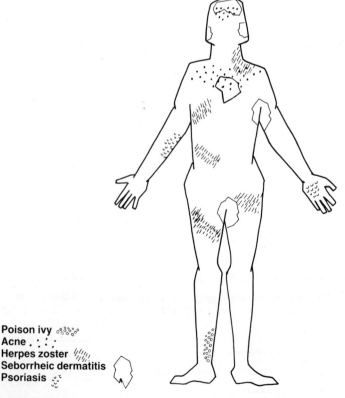

Poison ivy
Acne
Herpes zoster
Seborrheic dermatitis
Psoriasis

Figure 2–2. Characteristic location of common skin conditions.

    d. Configuration.

        (1) *Annular:* associated with drug reactions and psoriasis.

        (2) *Arciform:* associated with drug reactions and urticaria.

        (3) *Serpiginous:* seen in late syphilis.

        (4) *Iris grouping:* characteristically seen with erythema multiforme.

        (5) *Irregular:* associated with insect bites.

        (6) *Zosteriform:* characteristically seen with herpes zoster.

        (7) *Linear:* associated with contact dermatitis, particularly poison ivy.

3. Normal findings. Freckles on sun-exposed surfaces, single-to-multiple nevi, *keratosis,* especially in the geriatric client, and increased wrinkles in the elderly.

4. Clinical alterations (Fig. 2–2)

    a. Red, edematous skin commonly associated with acute skin disorders.

    b. Dry, thickened skin commonly associated with chronic skin disorders.

Primary lesion. Lesion that results from changes within the skin.

Secondary lesion. Lesion that results from change in the primary lesion owing to a continuing process.

To distinguish depth of skin lesion, note the following: skin slides over lesions below the dermis; skin moves with lesions within the dermis.

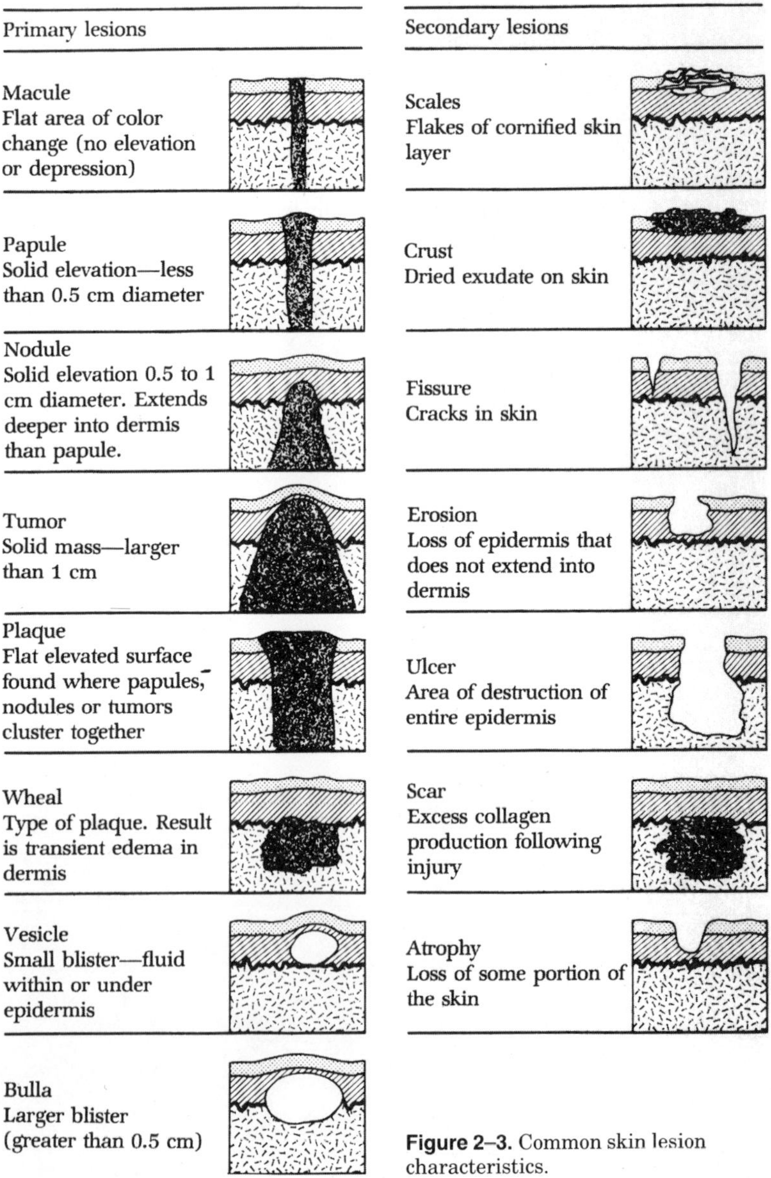

Primary lesions	Secondary lesions
Macule Flat area of color change (no elevation or depression)	Scales Flakes of cornified skin layer
Papule Solid elevation—less than 0.5 cm diameter	Crust Dried exudate on skin
Nodule Solid elevation 0.5 to 1 cm diameter. Extends deeper into dermis than papule.	Fissure Cracks in skin
Tumor Solid mass—larger than 1 cm	Erosion Loss of epidermis that does not extend into dermis
Plaque Flat elevated surface found where papules, nodules or tumors cluster together	Ulcer Area of destruction of entire epidermis
Wheal Type of plaque. Result is transient edema in dermis	Scar Excess collagen production following injury
Vesicle Small blister—fluid within or under epidermis	Atrophy Loss of some portion of the skin
Bulla Larger blister (greater than 0.5 cm)	

Figure 2–3. Common skin lesion characteristics.

IV. Palpation of the skin. Position client so that he or she is seated with involved skin areas exposed. Lightly palpate the skin using fingerpads of both hands to assess superficial or subcutaneous *primary* or *secondary lesions.*

   A. Detect masses or lesions on the skin or in the subcutaneous layers.

      1. Note size, shape, location, color, temperature, tenderness, depth,° and distribution.

      2. Normal findings. None. May find nevi, keratosis, or angiomas on the geriatric client.

      3. Clinical alterations (Fig. 2–3)

         a. Papule with shiny translucent border commonly associated with basal cell carcinoma.

         b. Large funguslike nodule commonly associated with squamous cell carcinoma.

         c. Blue-gray, irregularly shaped nevus often associated with malignant melanoma.

The body temperature varies with location, room temperature, season, activity, and state of anxiety.

Body temperature increases when the blood flow is increased to the skin area; temperature is decreased when the flow is reduced.

Lack of moisture in the axillary region is a key indicator of dehydration.

Dehydration is usually associated with furrowing of the tongue.

There is little excess skin overlying the sternum.

The depth of pitting edema should be measured in millimeters; it is no longer measured in terms of one to four plus.

B. Identify texture of skin.

 1. **Note** consistency.

 2. **Normal findings.** Soft and smooth, no lesions.

 3. **Clinical alterations**

    a. Velvety smooth skin often from hyperthyroidism.

    b. Rough, dry skin often from hypothyroidism or aging.

    c. Thickened skin commonly associated with chronic skin disorders.

C. Assess temperature of skin.°

 1. **Note** temperature of affected skin area.

 2. **Normal findings.** Skin warm to touch.

 3. **Clinical alterations°**

    a. Hyperthermia from inflammation, infection, burn, or fever.

    b. Hypothermia from cold exposure, shock, or decreased oxygenation.

D. Assess moistness of skin.

 1. **Note** dampness or dryness in various body areas, particularly the axillae,° groin, and skin folds.

 2. **Normal findings.** Moistness of skin varies among individuals; skin may be more moist in warm weather and dry in cold weather and in the geriatric client.

 3. **Clinical alterations**

    a. Excessive dryness often associated with dehydration,° myxedema, or diabetes.

    b. Excessive moisture associated with hyperthyroidism.

    Note: If signs of dehydration are evident, proceed to E. If not, proceed to F.

E. Assess turgor.

 1. **Technique.** Grasp skin over sternum between thumb and index finger,° release. Firmly press any areas of suspected edema with thumb.

 2. **Note** time it takes the released skin to resume its normal shape and depth of any pitting.°

 3. **Normal findings.** Skin immediately resumes previous shape, no pitting.

Pitting edema is not detectable until an adult accumulates 10 pounds of excess fluid.

Vascular areas are difficult to assess in dark-skinned persons.

Petechiae. Small, red hemorrhages.

Spider angiomas. Rare, small, deep red areas found below the level of the umbilicus.

Telangiectasis. Red, lacey dilatations seen in collagen-vascular disease.

Venous star. Bluish lesion with lines radiating from a central point.

The nails are an important indicator of the person's general health because they may be altered by disease. Therefore, they should be closely inspected.

The rate of growth of the nails varies with nutrition, age, and level of activity.

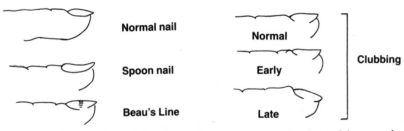

Figure 2–4. Abnormal curvature of the nails as compared to the shape of the normal nail.

Clubbing can be detected by the following changes:

   1. Increase in dorsel convexity

   2. Thickened, hard, and shiny nails

   3. Accentuated curve over free end

   4. Spongy atrophy of matrix

   5. Increase in angle of nail to 180 degrees

   6. Nail longer longitudinally than transversely

4. **Clinical alterations**

   a. Tenting associated with dehydration, rapid weight loss, or aging.

   b. Taut, shiny skin associated with the increased tension of edema.

   c. Pitting from excessive fluid often associated with congestive heart failure.°

F. **Detect areas of vasculitis.**°

   1. **Technique.** Diascopy: place slide over vascular area and press to blanch.

   2. **Note** any blanching or pulsations; color of surrounding area.

   3. **Normal findings.** None.

   4. **Clinical alterations**

      a. *Petechiae* fade but do not blanch.

      b. *Spider angiomas* blanch with pulsile center.

      c. *Telangiectasis* fades.

      d. *Venous star* fades.

V. **Inspection of the nails.**° **Position** client so that he or she is seated with hands on table; shoes and socks removed.

A. **Assess rate of growth.**°

   1. **Note** length of nails, pattern by history.

   2. **Normal findings.** Fingernails are completely replaced in 130 days; toenails in 1 to 1½ years.

   3. **Clinical alterations**

      a. Congenitally absent nails.

      b. Increased growth in warm weather, during increased activity and childhood.

      c. Decreased growth in cold weather, with lack of exercise, and aging.

B. **Assess curvature** (Fig. 2–4).

   1. **Note** angle of the nail in relation to the finger; shape.

   2. **Normal findings.** Dorsal convexity; 0 to 20+ degrees.

   3. **Clinical alterations**

      a. Platyonychia: flattening (hereditary)

      b. Koilonychia: spoon-shaped, fragile

      c. Rachet: wide, flat thumbnail

      d. *Clubbing:* increase in angle to 180 degrees with increase in dorsal convexity

Cyanosis of the nailbeds may be the first indication of the presence of cardiovascular disease.

Melonychia. Dark nails pigmented with melanin.

Assessment of grooming of nails is a good indicator of the client's self-image.

Biting of the nails is a habit and may be a clue to the level of anxiety or the addictive-type personality of the client.

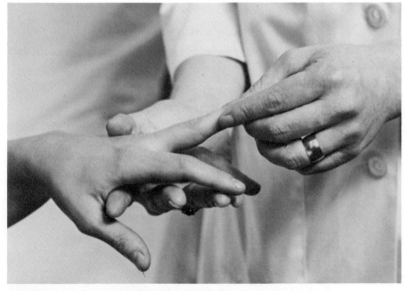

Figure 2–5. Palpation of the nails.

C. **Inspect color.**

1. **Technique.** Observe color; press nail firmly to blanch.

2. **Note** color and time in seconds for nail to return to normal color.

3. **Normal findings.** Transparent, pink with brown striae in black clients; color returns immediately when blanched (good capillary refill).

4. **Clinical alterations**

   a. Delayed filling from decreased circulation.

   b. Cyanosis from cardiovascular or respiratory disease.°

   c. *Melonychia* often associated with Addison's disease.

   d. Red lunulae associated with cardiac failure.

   e. Splinter hemorrhages running along the free margin associated with subacte bacterial endocarditis.

D. **Assess hygiene.**

1. **Note** grooming of nails.°

2. **Normal findings.** Clean, neatly trimmed nails.

3. **Clinical alterations**

   a. Dirty nails associated with poor personal hygiene.

   b. Bitten nails associated with anxiety.°

   c. Poorly trimmed nails from inability to groom own nails; often seen in the elderly, chronically ill and depressed clients.

VI. **Palpation of the nails. Position** client so that examiner holds his or her hand and systematically palpates each nail and nailbed (Fig. 2–5).

A. **Determine thickness.**

1. **Note** uniformity of thickness of the nail surface.

2. **Normal findings.** Uniformly thick.

3. **Clinical alterations**

   a. Increased thickness and dull, often associated with fungal infections.

   b. Decreased thickness from decreased peripheral circulation or anemia.

   c. Thickened, hard, and shiny nails associated with clubbing.

B. **Assess texture of the nail surface and matrix.**

1. **Note** uniformity of and consistency of the nail and nailbed.

2. **Normal findings.** Semitransparent, hard, smooth surface.

Beau's lines. Horizontal lines owing to the arrest of nail growth at the matrix.

Mees' lines. Longitudinal ridges on the nails.

3. **Clinical alterations**

   a. ***Beau's lines*** owing to infection, anemia, or malnutrition.

   b. ***Mees' lines*** associated with aging, anemia, infections, malnutrition, or arsenic poisoning.

   c. Spongy matrix associated with clubbing.

VII. Chart

A. **Skin.** Pink, warm, smooth, supple, elastic; freckles over sun-exposed area; clear, no skin or vascular lesions, discolorations, thickness, odor, or edema; good skin turgor; warm and moist to touch; mucous membranes pink and moist.

B. **Nails.** Pink, smooth, and hard; no biting, clean and well cared for; no clubbing or cyanosis; good capillary refill.

Assessment of the Head and Neck

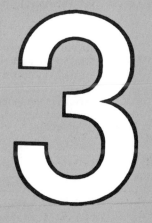

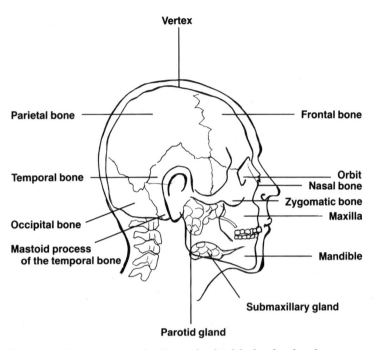

Figure 3–1. Bony regions and salivary glands of the head and neck.

Headache. A common manifestation of a variety of systemic problems, intracranial infections, tumors, and many disorders of the eye, ear, nose, and throat. Most clients who complain of headache usually suffer from migraines or muscle tension headaches. Muscle tension headaches are often associated with anxiety; they usually begin in the occipital area and spread "viselike" over the head. Migraines are often preceded by an aura and are typically unilateral. Headaches from brain tumors are usually progressive and recent in origin; this type of headache requires careful attention.

Diagnosis of the type of headache is usually made from a discussion of the signs and symptoms; physical signs are usually nonspecific.

Neck pain. Neck pain is a common complaint, but because of the vast number of structures in the neck, diagnosis can be difficult. Neck pain associated with stiffness usually indicates involvement of the muscles, bones, and joints of the cervical region. Neck pain associated with a cervical mass may be due to thyroid disease, lymphadenopathy, cysts, or tumors. Neck pain associated with swallowing or chewing often involves the pharynx, larynx, esophagus, salivary glands, or mandible.

I. Clinical considerations

A. A thorough knowledge of the anatomy of the head is essential (Fig. 3–1).

B. The examination of the head and neck includes inspection and palpation. Additionally, the neck is auscultated.

C. Inspection is vital when assessing the head and neck; unfortunately, simple observation is often neglected.

D. Examination of the head and neck is not difficult in the child because it does not require complicated maneuvers or instrumentation.

E. The fingerpads are more sensitive than the fingertips; therefore, they should be used to lightly palpate the delicate structure of the neck.

F. Any abnormal findings should be correlated to other systemic findings.

II. Relevant history questions

A. *Headache.* Ask questions related to the following:

1. Location, onset, quantity, duration, dispersion, character (throbbing or bandlike), pattern, and history of previous episodes or trauma.

2. Predisposing factors such as stress, menstruation, ingestion of alcohol, hypertension, hypoglycemia, medications, body position, or viral infection.

3. Associated signs and symptoms such as unilateral tearing, seizures, nausea or vomiting, constipation, visual disturbances, sleep disturbances, sensory changes, nuchal rigidity, or fever.

4. Use of therapeutic modalities.

B. *Neck pain.* Ask questions related to the following:

1. Location, onset, quantity, duration, dispersion, character, and history of previous episodes or trauma, thyroid disease or arthritis.

2. Predisposing factors such as trauma, anxiety, or strenuous physical activity.

3. Associated signs and symptoms such as headache, cervical swelling, fever, stiff neck, or numbness and tingling of the fingers.

4. Aggravating factors such as swallowing, chewing, or head and shoulder movement.

5. Use of therapeutic modalities, such as analgesics or cervical collars.

The size and shape of the skull vary with age, gender, and race.

The size of the head in adults should be in proportion to the size of the body.

Acromegaly. Bone overgrowth and thickening of the soft tissue caused by hypersecretion of the anterior pituitary hormones.

Microcephalus. An abnormally small head.

Hydrocephalus. An abnormally large head due to the accumulation of fluid in the subarachnoid spaces of the brain.

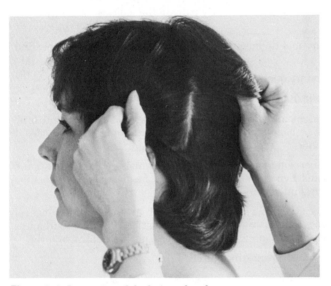

Figure 3–2. Inspection of the hair and scalp.

Sebaceous cysts. Round, smooth nodules formed from the plugging of sebaceous gland ducts. Cysts slide easily over the scalp.

Nits. Small, whitish-yellow eggs of lice, most often found at the nape of the neck. Nits adhere to a strand of hair; dandruff can be easily removed.

The face exhibits many racial and genetic variations.

Facial expressions reveal depression, anxiety, satisfaction, or embarassment.

The lips, nose, cheeks, ears, and oral mucosa readily show changes in color owing to aberrations of oxygenation.

III. Inspection of the head. Position client so that he or she is seated comfortably across from and facing the examiner.

    A. Inspect the skull.°

        1. Technique. Observe skull. Measure circumference at various intervals in children less than 2 years of age.

        2. Note size,° shape, symmetry, contour, and presence of lesions.

        3. Normal findings. Normocephalic skull size.

        4. Clinical alterations

            a. Deformities from trauma or head surgery.

            b. Enlarged salivary glands.

            c. Protrusion of the jaw owing to *acromegaly.*

            d. Thickened bones from Paget's disease.

            e. *Microcephalus* or *hydrocephalus.*

            f. Frontal bossing often from congenital syphilis or rickets.

    B. Assess condition of hair and scalp.

        1. Instructions to client. Remove any hairpiece or wig.

        2. Technique. Observe hair pattern. Hold blunt end of a cotton-tipped applicator and make vertical parts in the hair. Separate hair to expose scalp (Fig. 3–2). Repeat at 1-inch intervals, rotating around the scalp.

        3. Note color, texture, lesions, hair distribution, condition of scalp, hygiene, and presence of parasites.

        4. Normal findings. Clean, shiny hair; natural color. Hair is smooth in children; coarse in the geriatric client.

        5. Clinical alterations

            a. Greasy flakes from seborrheic dermatitis.

            b. Coarse, dry hair from hypothyroidism.

            c. Fine, silky, smooth hair from hyperthyroidism.

            d. Firm, nontender *sebaceous cysts.*

            e. *Nits.*

            f. Dirty or matted hair from poor personal hygiene.

            g. Alopecia from genetic factors or the aging process.

            h. Uneven distribution of hair in children often from chromosomal disorders.

    C. Inspect face.°

        1. Technique. Observe face in repose and throughout examination.

        2. Note symmetry, movement, expression,° color,° and condition of skin and any scars, lesions.

Orbital edema is often the first sign of the fluid retention associated with cardiac or kidney disease.

Myxedema. A deficit of thyroid hormone; hypothyroidism. Clients with myxedema have nonpitting edema, which causes the face to appear puffy.

Thyrotoxicosis. Toxic condition due to hyperactivity of the thyroid gland.

Cachexia. Sunken eyes, hollow cheeks, and dry, roughened skin associated with a severe debilitating disease or a state of starvation.

Salivary glands.

Parotids (in lateral cheeks)

Sublingual (under tongue)

Submandibular (under jaw)

The temporal artery is the only artery in the body that is normally tortuous.

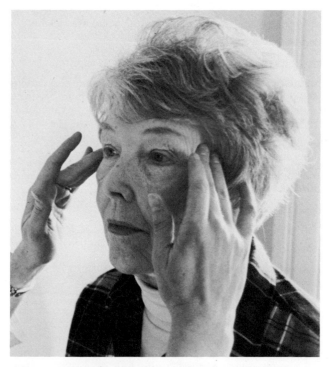

Figure 3–3. Palpation of the temporal arteries in the geriatric client.

Temporal arteritis. A chronic inflammatory disease that usually occurs in the elderly. There is throbbing pain in the temporal area with redness, swelling, and tenderness over the temporal artery. It is often accompanied by systemic symptoms.

3. **Normal findings.** Symmetric, alert expression, color the same as the rest of the body, soft texture and movement smooth.

4. **Clinical alterations**

   a. Periorbital edema from retention of fluid.°

   b. Cyanosis or pallor from changes in oxygenation.

   c. Jaundice from increased levels of bilirubin.

   d. Asymmetry associated with injury to the fifth or seventh cranial nerve or a cerebral vascular accident.

   e. Change in expression from mood or hormonal imbalances.

   f. *Myxedema* associated with hypothyroidism.

   g. Moon face and facial hair often from Cushing's syndrome.

   h. Loss of wrinkling of the forehead associated with **thyrotoxicosis.**

   i. Hollow face from **cachexia.**

   j. Multiple wrinkles often caused by excessive cigarette smoking.

   k. Bulging of lateral cheeks from enlarged **salivary glands.**

D. **Assess facial nerve (seventh cranial nerve) and trigeminal nerve (fifth cranial nerve) function.** (See Chapter 14, **III. D.** and **E.**)

IV. **Palpation of the head. Position** client so that he or she is seated comfortably across from the examiner. **Instruct** client to describe any tenderness.

A. **Palpate the temporal artery** in women over 40.

   1. **Technique.** Place fingerpads in both temporal areas. Simultaneously palpate temporal arteries, comparing one to the other (Fig. 3–3).

   2. **Note** character, consistency, and temperature of both temporal arteries.

   3. **Normal findings.** Slight pulsations in mildly tortuous arteries;° nontender.

   4. **Clinical alterations.** Warm, tender, cordlike artery often associated with **temporal arteritis.**

B. **Palpate scalp.**

   1. **Technique.** Gently palpate entire scalp, rotating fingerpads over skull.

   2. **Note** lumps or tenderness.

   3. **Normal findings.** None.

   4. **Clinical alteration.** Tenderness from lesions or cysts.

Mumps. A viral disease that causes pain and swelling of the parotid gland. Mumps vaccination is recommended as part of routine immunizations.

If mumps are suspected the orifice of the paratid duct (Stenson's) should be inspected for redness and swelling.

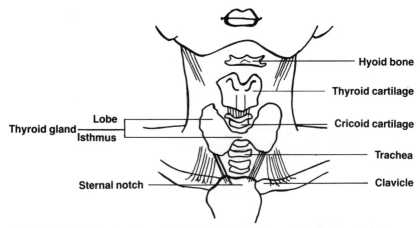

Figure 3–4. Anterior structures of the neck (sternocleidomastoid muscles partially shown).

Ankylosing spondylitis. A progressive form of arthritis causing ankylosis of vertebral joints.

Torticollis. Congenital or acquired stiffness of the neck caused by spasmodic contraction of neck muscles.

Tangential lighting. Lighting from behind to create a shadow. This type of lighting best reveals slight irregularities.

A glass of water enhances the client's ability to swallow repeatedly.

The thyroid is attached to the trachea and both rise with swallowing. Lymph nodes do not. The "Adam's apple" is composed of thyroid cartilage and is normally visible, particularly in men. It also rises with swallowing.

C. **Palpate the parotid gland in children.**

   1. **Technique.** Gently palpate in a line from the outer canthus of the eye to the pinna.

   2. **Note** lumps or tenderness.

   3. **Normal findings.** None.

   4. **Clinical alteration.** Tenderness from ***mumps.***°

V. **Inspection of the neck** (Fig. 3–4).

A. **Assess musculoskeletal function of the neck.**

   1. **Instructions to the client.** Point chin toward each shoulder. Then look straight ahead and look up at the ceiling, then down at the floor.

   2. **Technique.** Observe neck as client maneuvers head.

   3. **Note** position of head, movement, muscle development, symmetry, bulges, and visible pulsations.

   4. **Normal findings.** Neck is supple and rotates smoothly 90 degrees laterally and 70 to 80 degrees on extension. Client is able to flex chin on chest. Neck is midline; angle of jaw is equidistant from shoulders. Cervical spine is concave.

   5. **Clinical alterations**

      a. Stiffness and pain associated with cervical osteoarthritis or ***ankylosing spondylitis*** particularly in the geriatric client.

      b. Nuchal rigidity often associated with muscle tension or meningitis.

      c. Pain on motion from central nervous system disorders.

      d. Masses associated with thyroid disease, lymphadenopathy, or enlarged salivary glands.

      e. Asymmetry from ***torticollis*** or injury to the spinal accessory nerve.

B. **Inspect trachea and thyroid gland.**

   1. **Position of client.** Examiner faces client, who is seated. ***Tangential lighting*** may enhance inspection.

   2. **Equipment.** A glass of water.°

   3. **Instructions to the client.** Swallow a small amount of water when asked to do so.

   4. **Note** deviation of trachea, asymmetry of supraclavicular fossa, and unilateral or bilateral bulging of thyroid tissue as client swallows.

   5. **Normal findings.** Trachea is midline; thyroid tissue rises as client swallows.°

Palpation of the thyroid gland usually begins with the anterior approach because the client and examiner are already facing each other.

Tilting the client's head toward the side to be examined relaxes the sternocleidomastoid muscle and enhances palpation.

The firm placement of the examiner's hand on the client's shoulder provides leverage for the examiner and comforts the client.

The normal thyroid gland cannot easily be palpated. An enlarged thyroid gland rises under the examiner's palpating fingers as the client swallows. If anomalies of the thyroid gland are noted, other areas influenced by the thyroid gland (e.g., hair, skin) must also be assessed.

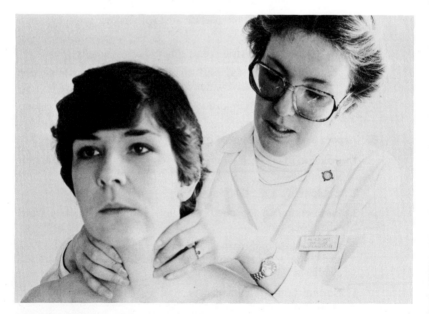

Figure 3–5. Posterior approach to the examination of the thyroid gland. (Note examiner displacing the thyroid gland to the left in order to palpate the left lobe.)

      6. **Clinical alterations**

          a. Deviation of trachea from masses, adhesions, lung disease, or neck surgery.

          b. Bulging of thyroid owing to goiter or nodules.

VI. Palpation of the neck

  A. Palpate thyroid gland using the anterior approach.°

      1. **Position** and **equipment.** See **V.B. 1** and **2.**

      2. **Instructions to client.** Slightly flex neck toward the side being examined.° Swallow when asked to do so.

      3. **Technique.** To examine the left lobe, place right hand on client's shoulder.° Grasp the sternocleidomastoid muscle with left hand, sliding thumb between the muscle and the tracheal cartilage to palpate lateral lobe. Ask client to swallow. Next release muscle and palpate surrounding area with fingerpads as client swallows again. Reverse procedure for right lobe.

      4. **Note** masses or nodules sliding under examiner's thumb as client swallows.

      5. **Normal findings.** Thyroid gland cannot easily be palpated, except in clients who have thin necks.°

  B. **Palpate thyroid gland using the posterior approach.**

      1. **Position.** Examiner stands behind client, who is seated. Client holds a glass of water.

      2. **Instruction to client.** Slightly flex chin toward chest. Swallow a small amount of water when asked to do so. Describe any areas of tenderness.

      3. **Technique.** Place fingerpads of both hands around client's neck. Palpate the isthmus by placing fingerpads in the midline of the neck, below the cricoid cartilage. Compare the right and left lobes by sliding fingerpads laterally, below the cricoid cartilage, on either side of the tracheal rings. Tilt head to the left and displace right lobe to the left (medially) with the right hand. Palpate the left lobe as client swallows using the fingerpads of the left hand (Fig. 3–5). Reverse procedure to examine the right lobe.

      4. **Note** motion of isthmus as client swallows. Compare lobes for size, contour, consistency, or tenderness as the client swallows again.

      5. **Normal findings.** Thyroid gland not usually palpable. The isthmus may be felt as a band of tissue that obliterates the tracheal rings. No nodules or enlargement of lobes should be felt.

Table 3–1. Manifestations of hyperthyroidism and hypothyroidism

Area affected	*Hyperthyroidism*	*Hypothyroidism*
Body movement	Frequent, fast	Slow, deliberate
Face	Alert expression	Dull, puffy
Emotional state	Labile, mania	Placid, depression
Voice	Normal	Coarse
Speech	Accelerated	Slow, distinct
Reflexes	Normal to hyperactive	Slow relaxation after response
Tongue	Fine tremors	Large and awkward movement
Skin	Soft and moist	Dry and thick
Hair	Fine, oily	Coarse and cracked
Nails	Onycholysis	Dry and brittle
Eye	Lid lag	Periorbital edema
Cardiovascular system	Tachycardia, atrial fibrilation	Bradycardia
Extremities	Pretibial myxedema	Thickened skin over dorsum of toes
Gastrointestinal system	Diarrhea	Constipation

Accessory nerve (less commonly called the spinal accessory). Innervates the motor portions of the trapezius muscle and the sternocleidomastoid muscle. Problems may be due to lesions or to injury at the base of the brain or in the cervical area.

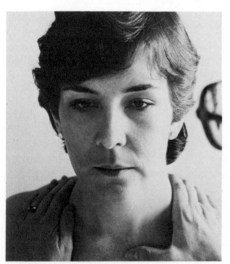 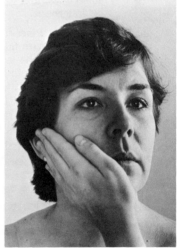

A   B

Figure 3–6. Assessment of accessory nerve (eleventh cranial nerve) function. A. Assessment of the function of the sternocleidomastoid muscle. B. Assessment of the function of the trapezius muscle.

6. **Clinical alterations** (Table 3-1)

   a. *Hyperthyroidism*

   b. *Hypothyroidism*

C. **Test function of the *accessory nerve* (eleventh cranial nerve)**

   1. **Position.** Client seated with shirt or dress removed so examiner can view neck and shoulders and scapular region.

   2. **Instructions to client.** Please push or pull against me when I ask.

   3. **Technique**

      a. Face client and observe position of head and shoulders.

      b. Place hand on client's forehead and ask client to bow head against resistance.

      c. Request client to turn chin to the right. Apply left palm to the left side of the client's chin and ask client to turn his or her head to the left and push away (Fig. 3–6A). Switch sides and repeat.

      d. Stand behind client and observe head and shoulders.

      e. Place both hands on client's shoulders and ask client to shrug against resistance (Fig. 3–6B).

      f. Ask client to spread arms out "like an airplane" and then move them up high.

   4. **Note** head position at rest; strength of neck muscles as head is flexed; the bulge of the sternocleidomastoid muscle as the head rotates to opposite side against resistance; level of both shoulders at rest; symmetry and strength of shoulder shrug; symmetry of scapulae as arms are raised horizontally; and presence of involuntary movements.

   5. **Normal findings.** Head is held in midline position; strength of neck and shoulder is symmetric; movements are smooth; and muscles are well developed.

   6. **Clinical alterations**

      a. Asymmetry from weakened sternocleidomastoid muscle.

      b. Shoulder droop or scapular rotation from weakened trapezius muscle.

      c. Muscle atrophy from injury to the eleventh cranial nerve.

Lymph nodes filter blood and form lymphocytes and monocytes to engulf bacteria. They enlarge in response to bacterial or viral infections.

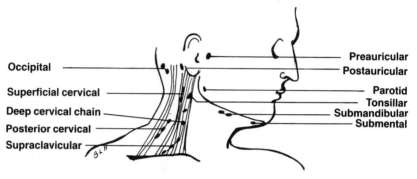

Figure 3–7. Distribution of the lymph nodes of the neck.

Hard, nontender nodes that are matted together are most often associated with metastatic disease.

Nodes that are soft, mobile, and tender often occur in response to an acute inflammation.

Bilateral lymphadenopathy in the neck is suggestive of systemic disease.

D. **Detect enlargement of *lymph nodes.***

   1. **Position.** Client seated facing examiner.

   2. **Instructions to client.** Try to relax and flex neck slightly forward or toward the side being examined. Describe any tenderness upon palpation.

   3. **Technique.** Gently rotate fingerpads allowing the skin to slide over underlying structures. Relax hands at all times. Bilaterally palpate the nodes in the following sequence (Fig. 3–7):

      a. **Preauricular.** In front of the tragus.

      b. **Postauricular.** Behind the auricle, on the mastoid process.

      c. **Parotid.** Over the parotid gland.

      d. **Tonsillar.** At the angle of the jaw.

      e. **Submandibular** (submaxillary). Under the side of the jaw.

      f. **Submental.** Under the mandible at the tip of the chin.

      g. **Superficial cervical.** Superficial to the upper portion of the sternocleidomastoid muscle.

      h. **Posterior cervical.** In the posterior triangle, behind the sternocleidomastoid muscle and anterior to the trapezius muscle.

      i. **Occipital.** Posterior base of the skull.

      j. **Deep cervical chain.** Under lower portion of sternocleidomastoid muscle.

      k. **Supraclavicular.** Above the clavicle.

   4. **Note** size, shape, mobility, consistency, temperature, and tenderness of nodes, and whether they are discrete or matted. If a node is enlarged, further explore the area it drains for any signs of inflammation.

   5. **Normal findings.** Nodes are usually not palpable. They may be felt as small, nontender, mobile nodes, especially in children.

   6. **Clinical alterations**

      a. Hard, fixed nodes often associated with metastatic cancer or lymphoma.°

      b. Tender, enlarged, mobile nodes often from an inflammatory process.°

      c. Lymphadenopathy associated with systemic disease.°

The client is instructed to hold his or her breath to eliminate breath sounds as the neck is auscultated for vascular sounds.

Hyperplasia of the thyroid gland causes increased blood through the thyroid arteries, producing vibratory sounds.

A venous hum is obliterated by lightly compressing the jugular vein.

VII. **Auscultation of the neck**

    A. **Instructions to client.** Be prepared to hold your breath when asked to do so.°

    B. **Listen for vascular sounds.**

        1. **Technique.** Place bell of the stethoscope over the carotid arteries, the subclavian arteries, jugular veins, and the thyroid gland. Listen for a few seconds at a time as client holds breath.

        2. **Note** equality and intensity of pulsations, presence of hums and bruits.

        3. **Normal findings.** None.

        4. **Clinical alterations**

            a. Carotid bruit associated with carotid stenosis.

            b. Thyroid bruit often from thyroid disease.°

            c. Venous hum.°

            d. Heart murmur radiating to the carotid arteries.

VIII. **Chart**

    A. **Head.** Normocephalic; full, even hair distribution; natural color; alert; no edema or uncoordinated movements; no lumps or tenderness; scalp clean, free of parasites.

    B. **Face.** Symmetric, no tics or periorbital edema.

    C. **Neck.** Midline position, full range of motion, smooth movements; thyroid gland nonpalpable, no nodes or bulges; carotids equal bilaterally, no carotid bruits or venous hums.

Assessment of the Mouth, Nose, and Sinuses

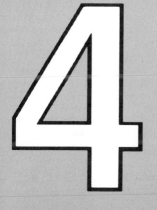

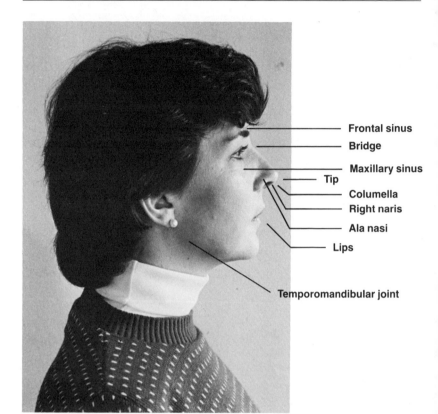

Figure 4–1. External anatomical landmarks of the mouth, nose, and sinuses.

Stomatitis. Inflammation of the buccal mucosa caused by pathogens, mechanical trauma, excessive use of alcohol, tobacco, or spicy food, vitamin deficiencies, or chemotherapy. Clinical alterations vary widely.

Pharyngitis. Inflammation of the mucous membrane of the pharynx or palatine tonsils. It usually accompanies a bacterial or viral upper respiratory tract infection. Less commonly, it may be caused by the ingestion of caustic liquids or the inhalation of toxic gases.

Rhinorrhea. Profuse, watery discharge often associated with an upper respiratory tract infection or allergies. Watery discharge is often indicative of a viral infection; a purulent discharge is usually caused by a bacterial infection. Cerebrospinal rhinorrhea occurs after a severe head injury and is usually unilateral. The discharge is usually clear but may be blood-tinged.

I. Clinical considerations

A. The examiner must possess a thorough understanding of the location of the anatomical landmarks of the mouth, nose, and sinuses (Fig. 4–1).

B. Assessment of the nose, mouth, and sinuses includes inspection and palpation of the nose and mouth, palpation and percussion of the sinuses, and auscultation of the temporomandibular joint.

C. Accurate and thorough examination of the mouth is essential; many examiners, however, are not sufficiently thorough.

D. The mouth should always be palpated using a glove or a finger cot.

E. Portions of the examination of the mouth and nose are uncomfortable for the client and are considered invasive. Procedures should be explained thoroughly.

F. The client needs to be aware that the examination of the teeth is not a substitute for a routine dental check-up.

G. A tongue blade should be used only when the client cannot depress and move his or her own tongue adequately.

II. Relevant history questions

A. *Stomatitis.* Ask questions related to the following:

1. Location, onset, quantity, character, pattern, duration, presence of lesions, and history of previous episodes.

2. Predisposing factors such as stress, smoking, poor dental hygiene, food, or change of seasons.

3. Associated signs and symptoms such as bleeding, ulcerations, or tingling.

4. Use of therapeutic modalities such as mouthwash or lozenges.

5. Dental check-up pattern.

B. *Pharyngitis.* Ask questions related to the following:

1. Location, onset, quality, quantity, pattern (enhanced by swallowing), duration, and history of previous episodes.

2. Predisposing factors such as exposure to toxic fumes, recent upper respiratory tract infection, or ingestion of caustic liquids.

3. Associated signs and symptoms such as fever, headache, earache, rhinorrhea, hoarseness, or voice changes.

4. Use of therapeutic modalities such as gargles, lozenges, or humidifiers.

C. *Rhinorrhea.* Ask questions related to the following:

1. Onset, duration, character of drainage, and history of previous episodes, nose or head trauma, or allergies.

2. Predisposing factors such as extensive use of nasal sprays, exposure to animals, change in seasons, or alcohol ingestion.

Epistaxis. A nose bleed. Epistaxis usually is due to external trauma to the nose, drying of the nasal mucosa with subsequent picking, or a nasal infection associated with vigorous blowing of the nose. Profuse bleeding without obvious cause warrants further assessment; blood coagulation disorders, hypertension, infections, and liver disease may all cause epistaxis.

Sinusitis. Acute sinusitis is a bacterial infection usually precipitated by a viral upper respiratory tract infection. It is considered chronic when the purulent discharge continues for more than three weeks. The sinuses are usually tender to palpation. Chronic sinusitis, however, may be asymptomatic.

The nose warms, humidifies, and filters inspired air.

The shape of the nose is primarily influenced by heredity and previous trauma.

Nasal *flaring.* Dilatation of nares during inspiration and constriction during expiration. It is usually seen with respiratory distress in the infant.

Nasal discharge is watery with allergies or viral infections; it is thick and purulent with bacterial infections.

The anterior two thirds of the nose is composed of cartilage; the posterior one third is bony. The nasal septum divides the interior nose into two separate air passages.

3. Associated signs and symptoms such as fever, lacrimation, sneezing, sore throat, postnasal drip, or nasal obstruction.

4. Use of therapeutic modalities, such as nasal sprays, antihistamines, or humidifiers.

D. *Epistaxis.* Ask questions related to the following:

1. Onset, pattern, duration, naris involved, character of discharge, and history of previous episodes or trauma.

2. Predisposing factors such as excessive use of aspirin, hypertension, easy bruising, nasal surgery, or recent upper respiratory tract infection.

3. Associated signs and symptoms such as pain, dizziness, nasal obstruction, or bleeding from other sites.

E. *Sinusitis.* Ask questions related to the following:

1. Location, onset, quantity, character, pattern, duration, and character of any discharge, and history of previous episodes, allergies, or upper respiratory tract infection.

2. Predisposing factors such as a recent upper respiratory tract infection.

3. Associated signs and symptoms such as fever, chills, yellow discharge, headache, or severe facial pain.

4. Use of therapeutic modalities such as steam inhalation, antibiotics, or nasal sprays.

III. **Inspection and palpation of the nose. Position** client so that he or she is seated comfortably.

A. **Inspect the external appearance of the nose.**°

1. **Note** skin surface, contour (profile),° relationship of nares to each other, and characteristics of discharge.

2. **Normal findings.** Color the same as facial skin, contour even, nares symmetric, no discharge visible.

3. **Clinical alterations**

a. Deformity from trauma or cleft lip.

b. Asymmetry of nares from obstruction.

c. *Flaring* or narrowing of nares with increased respiratory effort.

d. Copious or purulent discharge from rhinitis.°

e. Increased cartilage from acromegaly.

B. **Palpate the external nose.**

1. **Technique.** Place thumb and first finger on either side of the nose. Gently palpate from the bridge to the tip of the nose.

2. **Note** masses or tenderness and structure.°

Obstruction of both nares usually is due to rhinitis, nasal polyps, or an S-shaped deviation of the septum.

Aromatic substances such as mint, coffee, vanilla, lemon, and soap should be easy to identify. Sense of smell may be altered if inflammation is present or if the client has a history of allergy, heavy smoking, or head injury.

Anosmia. Loss of sense of smell.

Hyperosmia. An exaggerated sense of smell.

The brightness of the penlight in one naris transilluminates the opposite nasal passage.

    3. **Normal findings.** No masses or tenderness.

    4. **Clinical alteration.** Tenderness from internal or external lesions.

C. Test the patency of the nares.

    1. **Instructions to client.** Compress each nostril separately. Inhale and exhale through nose with mouth closed.

    2. **Note** flow of air through each naris.°

    3. **Normal finding.** Air flows unobstructed through nares.

    4. **Clinical alterations**

       a. Obstruction of one or both nares from a deviated septum.

       b. Mucosal swelling.

       c. Lesions.

D. Test the function of the olfactory nerve (first cranial nerve).

    1. **Instructions to client.** Close your eyes and compress each nostril separately. After testing, gently blow nostril.

    2. **Technique.** Dip a cotton-tipped applicator into an aromatic substance.° Place the tip under the client's opened naris.

    3. **Note** client's ability to detect and accurately identify common odors in both nostrils.

    4. **Normal finding.** Olfaction present bilaterally.

    5. **Clinical alterations**

       a. *Anosmia* from tumors or abscesses.

       b. *Hyperosmia* from hysteria, or inhalation or "snorting" of cocaine.

E. Inspect internal structures of the nose.

    1. **Position.** Client remains seated with head tilted back. A child should be held by an adult.

    2. **Equipment.** Nasal speculum with penlight or otoscope with speculum.°

    3. **Instructions to client.** You will feel pressure when the speculum is inserted but it will not hurt.

The blades of the speculum should be opened as wide as possible for optimum viewing of the turbinates.

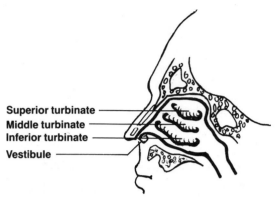

Figure 4–2. Internal structural cross-section of nose showing turbinates.

Avoid pinching nasal hairs as the speculum is removed by leaving the speculum open.

Kiesselbach's plexus. Area in the anterior, superior portion of septum containing superficial, small arteries and veins. This is the primary site of a nosebleed.

Turbinates. Bony shelves covered by vascular mucosa; they cleanse, humidify, and warm inspired air. The frontal, maxillary, and anterior ethmoidal sinuses drain into the middle turbinate.

The nasal mucosa is usually redder than the oral mucosa.

The nasolacrimal duct drains into the inferior meatus.

Folliculitis. Inflammation of hair follicles.

Polyps. Mobile, soft, pale gray overgrowths of mucosa found in the turbinates, usually seen in chronic rhinitis.

4. **Technique.** Place thumb on tip of client's nose. Gently push tip up and then back. Inspect nares. Close the blades of the speculum. With left hand grasp speculum between thumb and ring finger. Place index finger along upper handle and blade. Gently insert blades 1 cm into naris. Open speculum as wide as possible.° Stabilize speculum by placing left finger on client's ala nasi. Use right hand to hold flashlight and to maneuver client's head to best visualize the various parts of the nasal cavity (Fig. 4–2). Avoid any pressure on the tender septum. (An otoscope with a wide speculum may be substituted for the nasal speculum.) Remove speculum° and switch it to the opposite hand. Repeat with opposite naris.

5. **Note**

   a. **Mucosa.** Color, swelling, exudate, hydration, lesions, amount of hair, and condition of *Kiesselbach's plexus.*

   b. **Vestibule.** Lesions and amount of hair.

   c. **Nasal septum.** Presence of deviations, foreign body, lesions, or perforations.

   d. **Inferior *turbinate.*** Swelling, color, and exudate.

   e. **Middle turbinate.** Color, swelling, polyps or character, or any drainage from sinuses.

6. **Normal findings**

   a. **Mucosa.** Pink,° smooth, and moist, may be drier in the geriatric client.

   b. **Vestibule.** Small amount of coarse nasal hair.

   c. **Nasal septum.** Slight deviation or small spurs.

   d. **Inferior° and middle turbinates.** Pink, smooth, and moist. (The superior turbinate cannot be visualized with this technique.)

7. **Clinical alterations**

   a. **Mucosa.** Red and swollen owing to acute rhinitis; pale and boggy owing to allergic rhinitis.

   b. **Vestibule.** Fissures or *folliculitis.*

   c. **Nasal septum.** Deviation from trauma.

   d. **Turbinates.** Red and swollen from acute rhinitis; pale, blue-gray, and boggy from chronic rhinitis.

   e. *Polyps.*

Sinuses. Air-filled cavities lined with mucous membrane lying inside the bones of the skull. They become large enough to be palpated after a child is eight years of age.

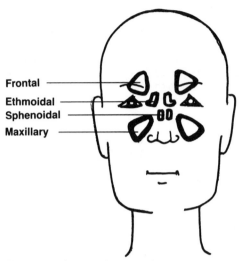

Figure 4–3. Anterior location of sinuses.

The shape and position of the lips are strongly influenced by genetic factors, the condition of the teeth, and the shape of the underlying bone.

The lips of dark-skinned persons contain more pigment. The many underlying vascular structures give the lips their reddish color.

The condition of the lips reflects pathologic variations within the body.

Herpes simplex. Also called cold sore or fever blister. They are small, painful vesicles which are commonly seen.

Rhagades. Linear periorbital scars.

Chancre. Large, indurated lesion found on the upper lip; site of initial entrance of *Treponema pallidum* in clients with syphillis.

Cheilosis. Ulcerations at corners of mouth.

F. **Palpate and percuss the maxillary and frontal** *sinuses* (Fig. 4–3).

   1. **Technique.** Directly percuss sinuses using middle finger to strike area. (Transillumination of the sinuses has limited use in a routine examination.)

      a. **Frontal sinus.** Place thumbs under bony ridge of eyebrow. Firmly press inward superiorly. Do not put pressure on eyeballs.

      b. **Maxillary sinus.** Place thumbs under cheekbones. Firmly press inward superiorly.

      c. **Sphenoidal** and **ethmoidal sinuses.** Not accessible for palpation or percussion.

   2. **Note** tenderness on palpation and percussion.

   3. **Normal finding.** No tenderness.

   4. **Clinical alteration.** Tenderness from acute or chronic frontal or maxillary sinusitis.

IV. **Inspection and palpation of the mouth. Position** client so that he or she is seated opposite the examiner throughout the entire examination of the mouth. Child is held securely by an adult.

A. **Inspect lips.**°

   1. **Instructions to client.** Please remove any dentures or prosthetics.

   2. **Note** shape, movement, color,° edema, contour, lesions, and state of hydration.

   3. **Normal findings.** Lips symmetric, smooth, pink, and moist.

   4. **Clinical alterations**°

      a. Vesicles from *herpes simplex.*

      b. Drooping or scar from cleft lip repair.

      c. *Rhagades* from congenital syphilis.

      d. *Chancre* from the initial infection of primary syphilis.

      e. *Cheilosis* from sun exposure, poor hygiene, or vitamin A therapy for acne.

      f. Cyanosis from decreased oxygenation.

      g. Pallor from anemia.

      h. Rodent ulcer from squamous cell carcinoma.

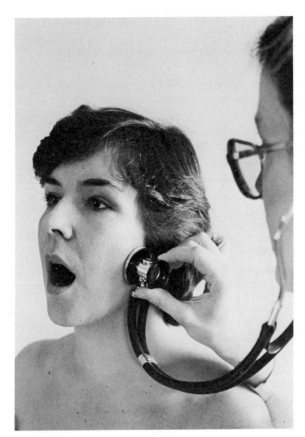

Figure 4–4. Auscultation of the temporomandibular joint for crepitus as client opens and closes her mouth.

Trismus. Inability to open mouth.

Myofacial pain dysfunction (MPD). Dull, preauricular pain; "clicking" sounds in the jaw commonly associated with tension-relieving clenching of the jaw.

Portions of the examination of the mouth may be momentarily uncomfortable for the client.

When palpating the buccal mucosa, push the outside of the cheek in between upper and lower teeth with free hand. This holds the mouth open, preventing accidental biting.

The oral mucosa has rapid healing capacity because of its increased vascularity. This ability is decreased in the geriatric client.

Stensen's duct. Opening to the parotid glands located adjacent to the second upper molars.

B. Palpate and auscultate temporomandibular joint.

1. **Instructions to client.** Open your mouth wide and then close it tightly. Describe any tenderness.

2. **Technique.** Simultaneously palpate both temporomandibular joints as client opens and closes mouth. Auscultate each joint as client opens and closes mouth (Fig. 4–4).

3. **Note** tenderness, crepitations, clicking, or limitation of movement.

4. **Normal finding.** Smooth, nontender movement of the jaw.

5. **Clinical alterations**

   a. *Trismus* or pain owing to tetanus.

   b. Arthritis of the temporomandibular joint.

   c. Trigeminal neuralgia or chronic anxiety.

   d. Pain from *myofacial pain dysfunction* (most common).

C. Inspect and palpate buccal mucosa.

1. **Instructions to client.** Hold mouth relaxed and partially open. Open wide when asked to do so.° Describe any tenderness.

2. **Technique.** Systematically inspect each area. Retract lips using both hands or two tongue blades. Use penlight to view all areas of the buccal mucosa as the opposite hand maneuvers the tongue, cheek, and lips with a tongue blade. Next, palpate all areas with gloved hand, holding the mucosa between thumb and index finger.°

3. **Note** color, lesions, texture, masses, tenderness, parotid gland secretions, and state of hydration.

4. **Normal findings.** Nontender, pink, smooth, moist mucosa.° Opening to *Stensen's duct* visible.

Leukoplakia. Patchy white plaques or spots on the mucosa.

Sjögren's syndrome. A connective tissue disorder that causes a defect in the secretions of the lacrimal and salivary glands.

Squamous cell carcinoma varies in appearance from erythema to ulceration. These cancers are extremely painful.

Candida patches can be peeled off, leukoplakia cannot.

Herpetic stomatitis (fever blister, cold sore) is an infection of the oral mucosa causing groups of vesicles containing clear fluid. Squamous cell carcinomas are usually ulcerated and extremely painful.

Fetor hepaticus. Musty odor similar to that of the excreta of mice, usually associated with hepatic coma from liver disease.

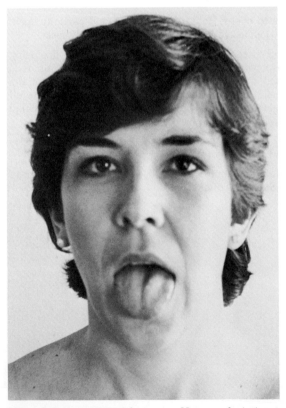

Figure 4–5. Inspection of the tongue. Note any deviation, tremors, or fasciculations as tongue is extended.

5. **Clinical alterations**

   a. *Leukoplakia.*

   b. Dry mucosa from dehydration or *Sjögren's syndrome.*

   c. Painful, ulcerative lesions, possibly from squamous cell carcinoma.°

   d. Dark pigmentation from Addison's disease.

   e. Small, curdlike patches from yeast infection (*Candida*).°

   f. Painful vesicular eruptions from herpetic stomatitis.°

D. **Assess odor of breath.**

   1. **Note** presence of any malodor.

   2. **Normal findings.** No odor present.

   3. **Clinical alterations**

      a. Fetor oris owing to poor dental hygiene.

      b. Sweet, fruity odor of acetone possibly from diabetic ketoacidosis or starvation acidosis.

      c. *Fetor hepaticus* seen in advanced liver disease.

E. **Inspect and palpate tongue** (Fig. 4–5).

   1. **Instructions to client.** First, tuck tongue behind lower front teeth. Then extend (to examine dorsum). Lift tip of tongue up against roof of mouth (to examine inferior surface). Move tongue to touch the inside of first the right cheek and then the left (to examine right and left lateral borders). Describe any tenderness.

If a client is unable to maneuver his or her tongue, a tongue blade may be used to depress and guide the tongue.

A white coating on the tongue is frequent and normal.

The tongue is an important diagnostic tool in the assessment of many diseases.

Congenital fissures run across the tongue; fissures owing to dehydration are longitudinal. A dry tongue from dehydration is usually accompanied by loss of skin turgor.

Xerostomia. Lack of saliva production seen in Sjögren's syndrome.

Hypoglossal nerve. The motor nerve to the tongue.

Fasciculations. Fine movements of the tongue when it is at rest.

Tremors. Fine movements of the tongue when it is protruded.

Dysarthria. Difficulty with articulation of speech.

2. **Technique.** Use penlight or otoscope as a light source as client completes maneuvers° described in **E. 1.** With gloved hand, palpate tongue between thumb and index finger.

3. **Note** color, size, coating, texture, ulcerations, lesions, and areas of tenderness.

4. **Normal findings.** Tongue pink° and moist. Rough papillae superiorly, with small veins sublingually.

5. **Clinical alterations**°

   a. Rough, dry tongue with longitudinal furrows often from dehydration.°

   b. Strawberry tongue from scarlet fever.

   c. Glossitis with brownish gray discoloration often from excessive smoking.

   d. Red, beefy tongue often from pernicious anemia.

   e. Marked indurations or painful ulcerations often owing to squamous cell carcinoma.

   f. Hairy, black tongue following prolonged antibiotic therapy.

   g. Large, lazy tongue related to slowed mental development.

   h. *Xerostomia* owing to Sjögren's syndrome.

F. Test *hypoglossal nerve* **(twelfth cranial nerve).**

   1. **Instructions to client.** Please open your mouth and move your tongue rapidly from side to side and then in and out. Say "Methodist Episcopal." Stick out your tongue.

   2. **Note** deviation of tongue to either side, *fasciculations, tremors,* and symmetry of shape. Note client's ability to say tongue twister.

   3. **Normal findings.** Tongue midline, no atrophy, no slurring of lingual speech, no fasciculations or tremors.

   4. **Clinical alterations**

      a. Deviation toward side of paralysis.

      b. Fasciculations seen in lower motor neuron disorders such as amyotrophic lateral sclerosis (ALS).

      c. Tremors often from thyrotoxicosis or anxiety.

      d. *Dysarthria* possibly owing to upper motor neuron disease such as multiple sclerosis (MS).

Tonsils. Lymphoid tissue that forms lymphocytes to fight bacteria, located on either side of the oropharynx. Scale for tonsil size is as follows:

Notation	Appearance of tonsils
1+	Only edges seen
2+	Edges seen midway between tonsillar pillars and uvula
3+	Edges extend to uvula
4+	Edges touch in midline

The size of the tonsils has little significance in determining the presence of chronic tonsilitis.

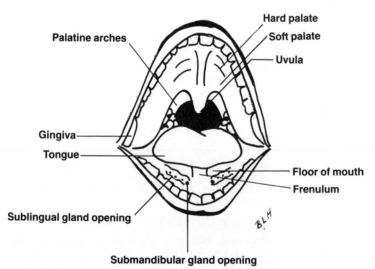

Figure 4–6. Structures of the mouth and the buccal cavity.

Ankyloglossia. "Tongue tied" from shortening of the frenulum.

G. **Assess function of the sensory component of the facial nerve (seventh cranial nerve) and the sensory component of the glossopharyngeal nerve (twelfth cranial nerve) for taste.** (See Chapter 14, III. F.)

H. Examine *tonsils.*

    1. Instructions to client. Hold mouth relaxed and opened wide. Tilt head back slightly. Say "Ahh" when asked to do so.

    2. Note presence or absence of tonsils, symmetry, color, size (see scale), shape, and presence of a membrane over tonsils.

    3. Normal findings.

        a. May or may not be present.

        b. Symmetric, pink (color of oral mucosa), and do not extend beyond tonsillar pillar.

        c. During childhood tonsils hypertrophy; they decrease in size after puberty.

    4. Clinical alterations

        a. Grayish abscess from tonsillitis.°

        b. Gray membrane covering tonsils owing to diphtheria.

        c. Peritonsillar abscess.

I. **Inspect and palpate the floor of mouth** (Fig. 4–6).

    1. Technique. Hold tongue to one side with the tongue blade. Shine a penlight onto the floor of the mouth. Palpate submandibular and sublingual salivary glands with gloved hand.

    2. Note color, lesions, and condition of frenulum and opening of ducts.

    3. Normal findings. Floor of mouth same color as oral mucosa; loose, pliable frenulum in center; firm, lobular opening of glands.

    4. Clinical alterations

        a. Indurated, painful lesions from squamous cell carcinoma.

        b. *Ankyloglossia.*

J. **Assess condition of teeth.**

    1. Instructions to client. This is not to be considered a substitute for a dental examination. Hold mouth relaxed and partially open.

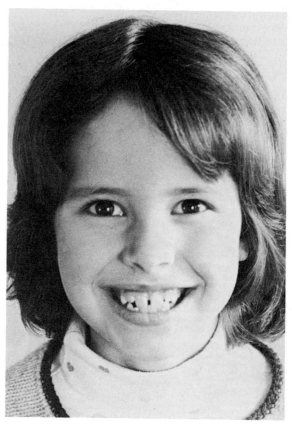

Figure 4–7. Eruption of lateral and central incisors in a 7-year-old child.

Table 4–1. Eruption of **permanent teeth**

Teeth	Age (years)
First molars	6–7
Central molars	7–8
Lateral incisors	7–8
First premolars	9–10
Second premolars	9–10
Canines	12–14
Second molars	12–14
Third molars	17–25

Vincent's stomatitis. "Trench mouth," small ulcerations covered by a gray-yellow membrane.

Lead line. Thin blue line in gums, 1 mm above margin of gingiva.

2. **Technique.** Count the number of teeth (Fig. 4–7). (May use a dental chart to record results.) Retract buccal mucosa laterally to aid in inspecting the teeth using tongue blade.

3. **Note** presence or absence of teeth; color, size, condition, shape, state of repair, and number of teeth; malocclusions; and use of prosthetics.

4. **Normal findings.** (Adult.) Thirty-two **permanent teeth** in good repair, ivory-white to yellow, upper teeth slightly overriding lower teeth. Number of permanent teeth varies with age (Table 4–1).

5. **Clinical alterations**

   a. Yellowed teeth from excessive smoking.

   b. Mottled enamel from excessive fluoride in water or tetracycline treatment.

   c. Caries or broken teeth from poor dental care. (More commonly seen in the elderly.)

   d. Moon molars owing to congenital syphilis.

K. **Assess condition of gums.**

1. **Technique.** Systematically inspect gingival tissue using tongue blade to retract buccal mucosa. Gently probe gums with cotton-tipped applicator.

2. **Note** inflammation or hemorrhage, retraction of gingival margins, and discolorations.

3. **Normal findings.** Shiny, firm, and pink gums; bluish with brown pigment in blacks; slightly receded gums in geriatric clients.

4. **Clinical alterations**

   a. Bleeding gums from inflammation (**Vincent's stomatitis**), traumatic brushing, or thrombocytopenia.

   b. **Lead line** from chronic lead exposure.

Gingivitis. Inflammation of the gums causing hypertrophy, not usually painful.

Pharynx

Nasopharynx: behind nose
Oropharynx: posterior from mouth
Laryngopharynx: posterior to pharynx

If the tongue blade is placed anteriorly, the tongue will arch up and cover the pharynx; the client may gag if the tongue blade is placed too far posteriorly.

Bacterial pharyngitis. Presence of exudate; cervical nodes are enlarged; pharynx is bright red; client has severe pain.

Viral pharyngitis No exudate; cervical nodes are enlarged; pharynx is dull red; client has mild pain.

Jaundice may first appear on the hard palate.

The vagus and glossopharyngeal nerves are tested together as they both supply motor and sensory function to the pharynx and larynx.

The uvula becomes red and swollen with inflammation of the pharynx or tonsils.

In bilateral paralysis there will be regurgitation through the nose when the client swallows and a nasal quality to the voice.

Glossopharyngeal neuralgia (throat pain) is rare.

       c. *Gingivitis* from periodontal disease.

       d. Cracked teeth and fillings from poor hygiene, more commonly seen in the elderly.

       e. Impacted molars in the adolescent.

L. **Inspect hard and soft palates and *pharynx.***

    1. **Instructions to client.** Tilt head as far back as comfortably possible.

    2. **Technique.** Place end of tongue blade in the middle of the arched dorsum of the tongue (cover two thirds of the tongue). Press down firmly by pushing thumb up against the middle finger, which acts as a fulcrum. Be careful not to pinch lower lip against the bottom teeth.°

    3. **Note** color, contour, exudate, and lesions.

    4. **Normal findings.** Hard palate is white to pale pink; soft palate is shiny, smooth, and pink.

    5. **Clinical alterations**

       a. High arch or perforation from cleft palate.

       b. Lesions or petechiae from ***bacterial*** or ***viral pharyngitis*** are more commonly seen in the school-aged child.

       c. Redness from inflammation.

       d. Jaundice from liver disease.°

M. **Test the function of the vagus nerve (tenth cranial nerve) and the motor component of the glossopharyngeal nerve (ninth cranial nerve).°**

    1. **Instructions to client.** Please open your mouth and say "Ahh." Be prepared to cough.

    2. **Technique.** Compress tongue as described in **K. 2.** Request that the client cough.

    3. **Note** symmetry of soft palate and uvula° and client's ability to cough.

    4. **Normal findings.** Symmetric rise of soft palate, no hoarseness or nasality, no difficulty swallowing. No deviation of uvula.

    5. **Clinical alterations**

       a. Failure of the soft palate to rise on one side; the uvula will be drawn to the normal side.

       b. Bilateral failure of the palate to rise.°

       c. Hoarseness owing to laryngeal swelling or paralysis.

       d. Severe throat pain.°

Note: The gag reflex is uncomfortable and should not be tested routinely unless there is hoarseness or uvular deviation.

Notes

V. Chart

A. **Mouth.** Lips symmetric, moist, no lesions, buccal mucosa pink and intact; hard and soft palates intact; tongue midline, no tremors or fasciculations; teeth in good repair; no gingival inflammation; no tenderness or crepitus at the temporomandibular joint; pharynx pink, no redness or exudate, uvula rises midline; tonsils present +2.

B. **Nose.** Straight, nares patent bilaterally; nasal mucosa pink and moist; no discharge or lesions, no tenderness, deformity, or perforations of nasal septum.

C. **Sinuses.** No tenderness.

Assessment
of the Ear

5

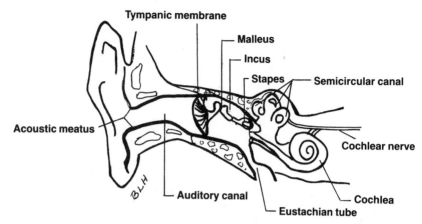

Figure 5–1. Internal structures of the ear.

Ear pain, or otalgia, may be due to a pathologic condition in the external or internal ear. Pain may also be referred to the ear from adjacent or distant sites. A sudden relief of severe pain is often due to the rupturing of the tympanic membrane and a subsequent relief of pressure. Ear pain is associated with most pathologic conditions of the ear.

Tinnitus. Tinnitus may be manifested as a continuous or intermittent ringing, buzzing, whistling, or roaring sound heard in one or both ears. Hearing loss is usually associated with it. The client usually complains that it is worse at night. Tinnitus may occur as a symptom of pathologic disorders of the ear, as a result of excessive exposure to noise, or from the use of ototoxic medications (may be the initial symptom of ototoxicity).

Hearing loss. Hearing loss accompanies many ear disorders, the use of ototoxic medication, and exposure to loud noise. Conductive hearing loss may be due to a lesion in the external auditory canal or the middle ear. Sensorineural hearing loss may be due to a lesion in the inner ear, cranial nerve damage, or it may occur as a normal part of aging. Hearing loss is often more evident to the client's family than to the client.

I. Clinical considerations

A. A thorough understanding of the anatomy of the ear is essential (Fig. 5–1).

B. The examination of the ear includes inspection and palpation of the ear and evaluation of hearing.

C. The client's response to simple directions is a good indication of his or her ability to hear.

D. The middle ear cannot be inspected; conditions involving the middle ear, however, are often reflected on the tympanic membrane.

E. A young child should be held by an adult during the otoscopic portion of the examination.

F. A tuning fork should not be struck forcibly because it will take too long for the tone to subside and the client may become impatient.

II. Relevant history questions

A. *Ear pain.* Ask questions related to the following:

1. Location, onset, character, quantity, duration, radiation, and history of previous episodes.

2. Predisposing factors such as swimming, airplane rides, exposure to cold, dental problems, recent upper respiratory tract infection, or allergies.

3. Associated signs and symptoms such as ringing, crackling, or buzzing in the ears, fever, dizziness, discharge, or difficulty in hearing.

4. Use of therapeutic modalities such as heat or analgesics.

B. *Tinnitus.* Ask questions related to the following:

1. Location, onset, character of the sound, duration, and history of previous episodes.

2. Predisposing factors such as excessive coffee intake, exposure to environmental noise, changing from one position to another, or use of ototoxic medications.

3. Associated signs and symptoms such as pressure, ear pain, hearing loss, or dizziness.

C. *Hearing loss.* Ask questions related to the following:

1. Onset, duration, specific tones or sounds not heard, and family history of deafness.

2. Predisposing factors such as chronic exposure to loud noise, ear infections, airplane rides, or use of ototoxic medications.

3. Associated signs and symptoms such as pain, tinnitus, dizziness, or discharge.

Otorrhea. Ear drainage may be associated with otitis externa, a ruptured eardrum, or a severe skull fracture. Drainage from the ear should be tested to determine the presence of cerebrospinal fluid. A foul-smelling discharge usually indicates infection. Brief, sanguineous fluid may be due to a ruptured furuncle or a perforated tympanic membrane.

Use of medications. Many drugs are ototoxic, affecting both the auditory and vestibular portions of the inner ear, particularly the organ of Corti. Temporary (from aspirin) or permanent (from streptomycin) hearing loss may occur. Because drugs are cleared by the kidneys, clients with renal failure are more susceptible to ototoxicity.

The *pinna* collects sounds and transports them along the auditory canal to the tympanic membrane.

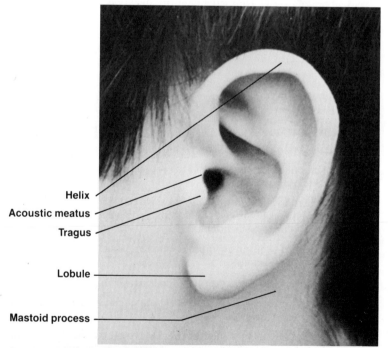

Figure 5–2. External structures of the ear.

Tophi. Pale, hard sodium urate crystals from chronic, long-standing gout.

Darwinian tubercle. Thickening along the posterior upper third of the helix.

D. *Otorrhea.* Ask questions related to the following:

1. Onset, duration, characteristics of discharge, and previous episodes.

2. Predisposing factors such as head trauma or recent ear infection.

3. Associated signs and symptoms such as pain, tinnitus, dizziness, or hearing loss.

E. *Use of medications.* Ask questions related to the following:

1. Recent history of ototoxic drug therapy (e.g., aspirin, streptomycin, gentamicin, neomycin, nitrofurantoin, kanamycin, and quinine).

2. Predisposing factors such as renal disease.

III. Inspection and palpation of the ear. Position client so that he or she is seated comfortably across from the examiner. **Instruct** client to be prepared to swallow when asked to do so and to describe any tenderness upon palpation.

A. Inspect the auricle or *pinna* (Fig. 5–2).

1. **Note** size, alignment, configuration, skin color, lesions, and discharge.

2. **Normal findings.** Ears symmetric, equal in size, the color of facial skin, with no lesions. Top of pinna aligns horizontally with corner of the eye. The verticle span of the pinna is less than 12 cm.

3. **Clinical alterations**

   a. Large ears associated with pernicious anemia.

   b. Reddened ears from capillary dilatation associated with a fever.

   c. Cyanosis of ears from decreased oxygen to the tissues.

   d. Congenital malformation associated with renal disease (oto-renal axis).

   e. Cardiac ear crease associated with atherosclerotic heart disease.

   f. *Tophi* caused by chronic gout.

   g. *Darwinian tubercle.*

   h. Skin ulcerations or cancers with prolonged exposure to the sun.

The pinna is rigid, composed mainly of skin and cartilage.

Acute otitis externa. Infection of the auditory canal, pinna, or both. Characterized by pain on movement of the pinna and tragus and a sticky yellow or purulent discharge from the canal.

Acute otitis media. Infection of the middle ear often accompanied by an upper respiratory tract infection. Symptoms include pain and impaired hearing. The incidence is greatest in childhood and decreases with age.

Obstruction of the auditory canal may be manifested by symptoms of deafness, tinnitus, or vertigo.

Foreign bodies are common in young children; odor is often the first symptom.

Furunculosis. Acute, tender, inflammation of hair follicles or sebaceous glands of the proximal third of the auditory canal.

Cerumen. Waxlike substance arising from the cartilaginous epithelium in the first third of the auditory canal. It traps foreign particles and acts as a lubricant.

Irrigation is contraindicated if the client has a history of otorrhea, perforation of the tympanic membrane, or recent head trauma.

Occlusion of the acoustic meatus with the tip of the irrigating syringe exerts too much pressure on the tympanic membrane because air is not allowed to flow back out.

Otoscope. A lighted instrument with a magnifying lens used to examine the auditory canal and the tympanic membrane. The following points should be kept in mind when using the otoscope:

1. Pull up and out on the pinna to raise the cartilaginous portion level with the bony portion. In children the canal is straightened by pulling down and out.

B. **Palpate the external ear.**

   1. **Technique.** Gently palpate pinna, bend forward, and pull on lobe.° Press on tragus and mastoid process.

   2. **Note** tenderness, swelling, lesions, consistency, and elasticity of the cartilage.

   3. **Normal findings.** Stiff pinna with no tenderness or lesions.

   4. **Clinical alterations**

      a. Tenderness of the tragus often from *acute otitis externa.*

      b. Tenderness of the mastoid process often from *acute otitis media.*

      c. Loss of sensation from dysfunction of the glossopharyngeal or vagus nerve (ninth or tenth cranial nerves).

C. **Inspect the acoustic meatus and the auditory canal°** (see Fig. 5–1).

   1. **Note** patency, odor, discharge, foreign bodies,° lesions, and inflammation.

   2. **Normal findings.** Lumen patent, skin pink and intact.

   3. **Clinical alterations**

      a. Otorrhea owing to infection or trauma.

      b. Excoriation of the walls of the canal often associated with *furunculosis.*

      c. Obstruction from a congenitally narrow lumen, *cerumen,* lesions, or a foreign body.

      Note: If you are unable to view the tympanic membrane because it is occluded by cerumen, and if no signs or symptoms indicate perforation, proceed to section D.

D. **Remove any excess cerumen from auditory canal.°**

   1. **Instructions to client.** Lie on your side on your unaffected ear. You may feel slight pressure and dizziness as the solution is being instilled into your ear.

   2. **Technique.** Fill an ear syringe with warmed and diluted hydrogen peroxide and gently instill into the acoustic meatus. Do not occlude the meatus with the tip of the syringe.° Direct flow upward; do not aim directly at the tympanic membrane. Allow solution to soak for 5 minutes and then repeat procedure and rinse with warmed tap water. Gently swab dry any accessible portions of the external ear.

E. **Insert *otoscope* into the auditory canal, view the tympanic membrane.**

   1. **Position.** Client is seated comfortably with head bent toward the opposite side to be examined. Child is held by an adult.

2. Use the largest speculum possible that fits comfortably in the canal for maximum visualization of the tympanic membrane and decreased manipulation of the scope.

3. Rotate otoscope while inserting to prevent scraping the sensitive canal walls.

4. The epithelium lining the proximal canal is sensitive because it is stretched over bone.

5. Arnold's nerve is a branch of the vagus and is located in the auditory canal; stimulating it as the speculum is inserted may cause the client to cough.

6. The right ear should be examined with the otoscope in the examiner's right hand; the left ear, with the otoscope in the examiner's left hand.

7. Portions of the tympanic membrane may be obscured by the auditory canal; the position of the otoscope must be changed to view all aspects.

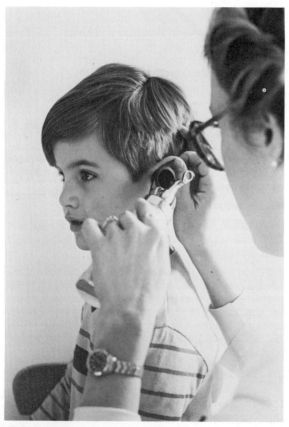

Figure 5–3. Otoscopic examination of the tympanic membrane in the child. Notice how the examiner pulls out and down.

2. **Instructions to client.** You may feel pressure that causes you to cough as the otoscope cone is inserted.

3. **Technique**

   a. **Right ear.** Grasp upper portion of the pinna between thumb and index finger of the left hand. Be careful not to dig into client's ear with your fingernails. Pull the flexible cartilage upward and outward in the adult, downward in the child. Steady client's head. Lightly hold the otoscope between thumb and middle finger of your right hand. Initially hold the otoscope parallel to the canal and gently insert into the meatus. Slowly rotate otoscope downward while progressing into the canal. Once the membrane has been visualized, vary position to view all aspects. Keep pinna retracted and reverse procedure to withdraw speculum.

   b. **Left ear** (Fig. 5–3). Lightly grasp left ear with your right hand. Insert speculum with your left hand, using the technique described in **E. 3.** (Examining the left ear is often difficult for the examiner who is right-handed, and vice versa.)

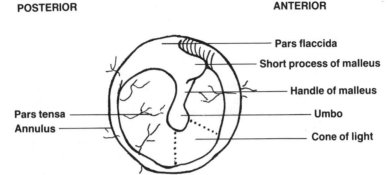

Figure 5–4. Landmarks of the right tympanic membrane.

In the adult, the auditory canal is 2.5 cm long. The first third is cartilaginous and curves up and forward; the inner two thirds curves posteriorly through the temporal bone. The auditory canal is horizontal in the child.

Serous otitis media. Accumulation of sterile fluid in the middle ear secondary to obstruction of the eustachian tube. It often follows an upper respiratory infection or an airplane ride. Symptoms include pain and ears feeling plugged.

Barotrauma. Rupture of the tympanic membrane and bleeding into the middle ear caused by an increase in atmospheric pressure, which exerts pressure directly on the tympanic membrane.

Meniscus. Line of fluid seen on the tympanic membrane. It is most commonly associated with serous otitis media.

Obstruction of the eustachian tube causes a negative pressure to build up behind the tympanic membrane, causing it to retract. Fluid is then drawn from surrounding tissue, creating a meniscus.

Forceful exhalation may exert too much pressure on the tympanic membrane and cause pain.

The tympanic membrane will bulge outward as the air is trapped within the upper airway.

The **eustachian tube** is located between the pharynx and the middle ear. It equalizes pressure on either side of the tympanic membrane and is normally closed except during yawning or swallowing.

Human speech ranges from 300 to 3000 hertz (Hz), or cycles per second.

4. **Note the following** (Fig. 5–4).

   a. Bulging: landmarks are obscured.

   b. Retraction: landmarks are more prominent.

   c. Cone of light: distorted, diffuse, or spotty.

   d. Sheen and thickness of membrane.

   e. Perforations: usually found just inside the annulus.

   f. Vascularity.

5. **Normal findings.**° Intact, shiny, pearly gray membrane (may dull with age). Cone of light at the 5 o'clock position in the right ear and at the 7 o'clock position in the left ear. (Cone of light is slightly more diffuse in children.) Membrane pulled slightly inward at the center (umbra).

6. **Clinical alterations**

   a. Bulging of the tympanic membrane from fluid, pus, or blood in the middle ear. Pus is often associated with acute otitis media.

   b. Retraction from blockage of the eustachian tube often associated with **serous otitis media.**

   c. Discolorations

      (1) Amber or yellow from serum.

      (2) Chalky white from pus.

      (3) Blue from blood often from **barotrauma.**

   d. **Meniscus** from fluid.°

F. **Test mobility of the tympanic membrane.**

   1. **Equipment.** Otoscope. Use a pneumatic otoscope for a child or a client who is unable to follow directions.

   2. **Instructions to client.** Pinch nose, close mouth, and exhale gently.°

   3. **Note** (with otoscope in place) mobility of the tympanic membrane as client breathes.

   4. **Normal findings.** Membrane bulges outward° from the increase in pressure within the **eustachian tube.**

   5. **Clinical alterations.** Loss of mobility from perforation or scar.

G. **Measure ability to hear whispered voice.**°

   1. **Position.** Examiner stands behind client, 1 to 2 feet from ear. (Examiner may remain in front of client and have him or her close both eyes to prevent lipreading.)

   2. **Instructions to client.** Occlude ear not being tested by placing your finger in acoustic meatus. Wiggle finger to mask environmental noises. Immediately repeat words or numbers heard.

Whispered sounds are higher-pitched than the normal speaking voice.

Hearing should always be tested in one ear at a time.

The development of normal speech patterns in children is a positive indication of the child's ability to hear.

Conductive hearing loss from otosclerosis is responsible for 50 percent of all deafness in persons more than 50 years of age.

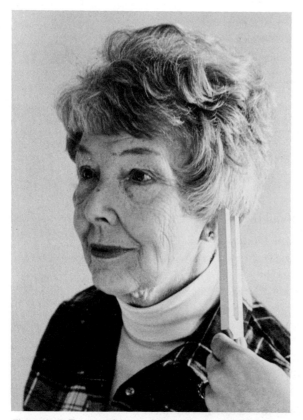

Figure 5–5. Testing of air conduction during the Rinne test.

Conductive hearing loss. Interpretation of the transmission of vibrations from the external ear to the cochlea. The client hears well through bone conduction. The Rinne test will be negative. The Weber test will lateralize to the affected ear.

3. **Technique.** Whisper simple words or numbers into ear to be tested.° (Exhale first to decrease the intensity of your voice.) Vary tones used to test client's ability to hear different frequencies. Repeat procedure for opposite ear.° (May hold a ticking watch 1 to 2 inches from ear to test higher-pitched sounds.)

4. **Note** client's ability to accurately repeat whispered words or numbers.

5. **Normal findings.** Client is able to repeat all sounds heard in both ears. This ability may decrease in clients more than 50 years of age.°

6. **Clinical alterations.** Hearing loss from otosclerosis,° chronic ear infections, environmental exposure to loud noise, use of ototoxic drugs, or birth defects (maternal rubella).

H. **Compare bone conduction to air conduction—Rinne test;** (Fig. 5–5).

1. **Position.** Client seated directly opposite the examiner.

2. **Equipment.** Tuning fork, 512 or 1024 Hz. Set fork in motion by lightly striking palm.

3. **Instructions to client.** Raise hand when vibrations are no longer heard. Nod head when they resume.

4. **Technique.** Place handle of vibrating fork on the mastoid process to test bone conduction. Be careful not to touch client's hair. When client signals that the sound is no longer heard (not felt), quickly bring prongs around to the acoustic meatus to test air conduction. Be careful not to touch client and dampen vibrations. Record time client hears sound in seconds.

5. **Note** the length of time of bone conduction (when the fork is on the mastoid process) in comparison to air conduction (when the fork is in front of the acoustic meatus).

6. **Normal findings.** Air conduction is twice as long as bone conduction, or Rinne positive. AC–2; BC–1 bilaterally.

7. **Clinical alterations.** Air conduction equal to or less than bone conduction, or Rinne negative. This finding may be associated with a *conductive hearing loss.*

I. **Test for lateralization of sound (Weber test).**

1. **Position and equipment.** See **H. 1** and **2.**

2. **Instructions to client.** Point to the ear in which you hear the sound the loudest.

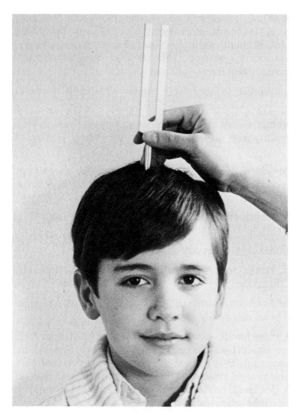

Figure 5–6. The Weber test: Proper placement of the tuning fork when testing for lateralization of sound.

Sensorineural hearing loss. Loss of perceptive hearing because of a defect in the inner ear or auditory nerve (eighth cranial nerve). The Rinne test will be positive, and the Weber test will lateralize to the better hearing ear.

3. **Technique.** Place handle of vibrating tuning fork on the top (vertex) of the client's head in the midline (Fig. 5–6).

4. **Note** sensorineural or conductive hearing loss (which ear the client identifies as hearing the sound best).

5. **Normal finding.** Sound heard equally well in both ears.

6. **Clinical alterations**

   a. Conductive loss (air conduction): lateralization to the side of the poorer hearing ear. (Environmental noises are not conducted through the canal, only through the bone.)

   b. Sensorineural loss: lateralization to the better hearing ear because the cochlea is functioning effectively.

J. **Perform the Schwabach test to confirm the presence of a *sensorineural hearing loss.***

   1. **Instructions to client.** Nod if you still hear the sound from the tuning fork.

   2. **Technique.** Quickly alternate vibrating tuning fork between examiner's ear and the client's ear. When client no longer signals that he or she hears the sound, quickly return tuning fork to examiner's own ear.

   3. **Note** the continuation of any sound heard by you, the examiner.

   4. **Normal findings.** Assuming that you, the examiner, have normal hearing, the sound from the vibrations should cease when they cease for the client.

   5. **Clinical alterations.** If the examiner hears the sound, the client may have a sensorineural loss.

K. **Vestibular testing.** See Chapter 14, **V. B.**

IV. **Chart**

A. **Ear.** Symmetric bilaterally, no deformities, masses, or discharge; no erythema or edema of auditory canal; no ceruminosis; tympanic membrane pearly-gray and translucent; negative perforations, swelling or retraction; light reflex present.

B. **Hearing.** Hears whispered voice bilaterally; Rinne positive bilaterally AC>BC; equal lateralization; Schwabach negative.

Assessment
of the Eye

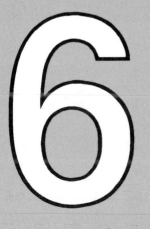

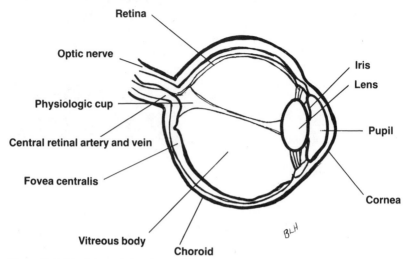

Figure 6–1. The internal structures of the eye.

Pain in the eye is important and demands thorough investigation. Serious causes include uveitis and acute glaucoma. Obvious local causes include infection, injury, and a foreign body concealed beneath the upper lid. Eye pain may be referred (i.e., sinusitis). Simple eye discomfort often indicates eyestrain from close or prolonged reading.

Alterations in vision are commonly seen with simple refractive errors, corneal opacities, cataracts (particularly in the older diabetic), macular degeneration (particularly in the geriatric client), optic neuritis, and optic atrophy. A sudden change in vision should be considered an emergency. Most conditions can be correctly diagnosed by a complete history and examination of specific manifestations.

I. General considerations

A. The examiner must possess a thorough understanding of the anatomy and physiology of the eye (Fig. 6–1).

B. Examination of the eye includes inspection and palpation of the anterior structures of the eye, the testing of visual acuity, extraocular movements, peripheral vision, the assessment of PERRLA (*p*upils *e*qual, *r*ound, *r*eact to *l*ight, and *a*ccommodation), and the ophthalmoscopic examination.

C. The ophthalmoscopic examination is necessary to view the internal structures of the eye, the lens, vitreous, and retina.

D. Examination of the eye should always be included as part of a routine physical examination because there are many ocular manifestations of systemic disease.

E. The examination room should provide bright lighting for inspection and reduced lighting for the ophthalmolscopic examination.

F. When the client is asked to direct his or her gaze at a target object, either the examiner's finger or a penlight (which may or may not be lit) should be used.

II. Relevant history questions

A. Eye pain.° Ask questions related to the following:

1. Onset (sudden or gradual), location (one or both eyes), duration, pattern, radiation (to teeth or ears), quantity, quality, history of recent trauma to the head or eye, recent febrile illness, previous episodes, and pertinent family history.

2. Predisposing factors such as eyestrain, constipation, stress, corrective lenses, exposure to environmental irritants, or changing from one position to another.

3. Associated signs and symptoms such as headache, fever, altered vision, increased lacrimation, or feeling pressure behind the eye.

B. Alteration in vision.° Ask questions related to the following:

1. Onset (sudden or gradual), location (one or both eyes), duration, pattern (day or night disturbances), character (blurred vision, photophobia, spots), history of recent trauma, febrile illness, previous episodes, and pertinent family history.

2. Predisposing factors such as age, diabetes, refractive errors, stress, or exposure to environmental irritants.

3. Associated signs and symptoms such as headache, eye pain, fever, increased lacrimation, pressure behind the eye, or fatigue.

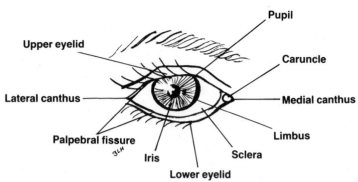

Figure 6–2. Anatomy of the eye, anterior view.

The skin of the eyelids is the thinnest skin on the body. Thin strips of connective tissue (tarsal plates) give the eyelids their consistency.

Hordeolum (stye). Inflammation of a sebaceous gland leading to the formation of a pustule on the lid margin.

Ptosis. Drooping of the eyelids.

Xanthelasma. Wartlike, raised yellow plaque, often found on lids near canthi.

Exophthalmos. Forward protrusion or bulging of the eyeball, commonly associated with Graves' disease.

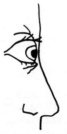

Figure 6–3. Exophthalmos.

III. **Inspection of the eyes** (Fig. 6–2). **Position** client so that he or she is seated comfortably in a well-lit room. **Instruct** client to keep his or her eyes open naturally and to relax and look straight ahead.

A. **Inspect the eyebrows.**

1. **Note** distribution, color, and condition and quality of hair.

2. **Normal findings.** Eyebrows fully distributed, color same as hair, thicker and coarser in the geriatric client, particularly men.

3. **Clinical alterations**

   a. Loss of lateral third of eyebrows commonly associated with thyrotoxicosis.

   b. Scaliness owing to seborrhea.

B. **Inspect the eyelids.**°

1. **Note** color, shape, symmetry, edema, lesions, and scaliness.

2. **Normal findings.** Intact, smooth skin covering 2 to 3 mm of cornea, lids open and close easily with some excess skin in the geriatric client.

3. **Clinical alterations**

   a. *Hordeolum* from infection of a meibomian gland of the eyelid.

   b. *Ptosis* congenitally acquired or from oculomotor nerve paralysis in myasthenia gravis.

   c. *Xanthelasma* commonly associated with hypercholesteremia.

C. **Test for lid lag.**

1. **Instructions to client.** Follow my finger as rapidly as possible.

2. **Technique.** Hold finger 20 inches (8 cm) above client's head. Rapidly move finger down.

3. **Note** ability of the upper lid to follow the downward movement of the iris.

4. **Normal findings.** Lid overlaps iris as eyes close.

5. **Clinical alterations.** Movement of the lid lagging behind, exposing a white area of sclera commonly associated with *exophthalmos* (Fig. 6–3).

D. **Inspect the eyelashes.**

1. **Note** direction of lashes, exudate, erythema, and scaling.

2. **Normal findings.** Eyelashes clean and full; fewer hairs in the geriatric client.

Entropion. Inward turning of the lid and lashes, causing irritation of the conjunctiva.

Ectropion. Outward turning of the lid and lashes.

Blepharitis. Reddened lid margins with flaking and scaling.

The lacrimal gland lubricates and cleanses the conjunctiva and cornea.

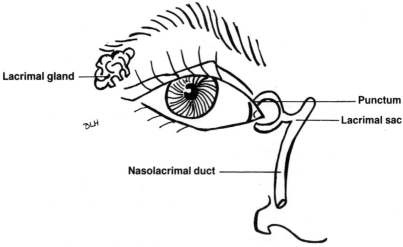

Figure 6–4. Lacrimal apparatus.

The **sclera** is covered and protected by the bulbar conjunctiva; the palpebral conjunctiva lines the inside of the eyelids.

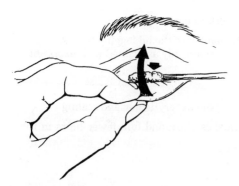

Figure 6–5. Technique of eversion of the eyelid.

3. **Clinical alterations**

   a. *Entropion.*

   b. *Ectropion.*

   c. *Blepharitis.*

E. **Inspect and palpate the lacrimal apparatus of the eye.**°

   1. **Technique.** Place finger over lacrimal sac and apply firm pressure (Fig. 6–4). Press area under punctum lacrimale.

   2. **Note** any discharge from punctum and consistency of lacrimal gland.

   3. **Normal findings.** No discharge; tissue of lacrimal gland smooth.

   4. **Clinical alterations**

      a. Constant tearing or the expression of fluid from punctum from an obstructed duct.

      b. Redness and swelling of the punctum caused by infection of the lacrimal duct.

      c. Lack of adequate tearing.

F. **Assess *sclera* and palpebral and bulbar conjunctiva** (Fig. 6–5).

   1. **Instructions to the client.** I need to pull your upper lid back. It may feel uncomfortable but it will not hurt you. When the lid is retracted, look up, down, and to each side. When the lower lid is retracted, look upward.

   2. **Technique**

      a. **Upper lid.** Gently grasp lashes between thumb and forefinger. Gently pull down and out. Place the plain end of a cotton-tipped applicator above the lid margin. Using the stick as a fulcrum, firmly fold eyelid over the applicator, everting the lid. Hold the lid inside out by anchoring the lashes against the bony orbit. When inspection is complete, gently unfold the lid and allow eyelid to fall back in place as client looks up. Use the right hand to retract lid when examining the left eye, and vice versa.

      b. **Lower lid.** Place both thumbs below eyes, on the infraorbital margin. Displace skin down, exposing the sclera and conjunctiva.

   3. **Note** color, swelling, lesions, moistness, and clarity as client moves eye.

   4. **Normal findings.** Shiny, china-white sclera covered by moist, shiny, transparent bulbar conjunctiva. A bluish hue may be seen in the elderly. Spots of brown melanin may be seen, varying with race. Palpebral conjunctiva is pink and intact.

Pinguecula. Raised yellow triangular plaques on each side of the limbus. The larger one is usually on the nasal side.

Pterygium. A triangular growth of vacularized conjunctiva, extending from the nasal canthus toward the cornea.

Cornea. Protective covering of the pupil and the iris.

Corneal abrasions. Painful scratches on the cornea, which should be stained to be detected accurately. Staining is not a routine procedure.

Arcus senilis. Bilateral gray bands surrounding the cornea, most commonly seen in the black geriatric client.

Iris. A circular, colored structure that contains two muscles that regulate its size, depending on light available and distance of object viewed.

Brushfield's spots. Darkly pigmented areas in the iris.

Ciliary flush. Congestion of the vessels of the iris producing a red band around the limbus.

Coloboma. A cleft or fissure in the iris.

Corneal reflex. Blinking of the eyes when the ophthalmic branch of the trigeminal nerve is stimulated.

Blinking is due to the corneal reflex; tearing is caused by the irritation from the cotton.

5. **Clinical alterations**

   a. Yellow sclera associated with jaundice.

   b. *Pinguecula* often from chronic exposure to irritants.

   c. *Pterygium* often from chronic exposure to irritants.

   d. Pale palpebral conjunctiva commonly associated with anemia.

   e. Inflammation of the bulbar conjunctiva owing to a bacterial or viral infection or an allergic response.

G. **Inspect the *cornea* and lens.**

   1. **Instructions to the client.** Look directly ahead.

   2. **Technique.** Shine penlight obliquely across each cornea.

   3. **Note** opacities, scars, and superficial irregularities.

   4. **Normal findings.** Smooth, moist, and transparent cornea.

   5. **Clinical alterations**

      a. *Corneal abrasions* associated with trauma or use of contact lenses.

      b. *Arcus senilis.*

      c. Dullness usually associated with glaucoma or chronic nutritional deficiencies.

H. **Inspect the *iris.***

   1. **Note** color, shape, and clarity.

   2. **Normal findings.** Round, flat pigment varies with genetic influences; *Brushfield's spots.*

   3. **Clinical alterations**

      a. Bulging of iris toward cornea.

      b. *Ciliary flush.* Associated with inflammation of the iris.

      c. *Coloboma.*

I. **Elicit *corneal reflex.***

   1. **Equipment.** Wisp of cotton fiber twisted from a cotton-tipped applicator.

   2. **Instructions to client.** Your eye will be touched very lightly. Try to keep your eyes open, it will not hurt.

   3. **Technique.** Lightly touch cornea with cotton; repeat in opposite eye.

   4. **Note** symmetric blinking of both eyes, tearing in the eye touched.°

   5. **Normal findings.** Lids of both eyes blink when either eye is touched.

Hirschberg's test. Corneal light reflex.

Amblyopia. Reduced vision owing to the disuse of a structurally normal eye. Screening children less than 6 years of age is essential to avoid permanent blindness.

Pupils reach maximum size in early adulthood and become progressively smaller with age.

Seventy-five percent of the population has even pupils and twenty-five percent has uneven pupils. This statistic must be recorded as baseline data.

Anisocoria. Uneven pupils.

Mydriasis. Dilated pupils.

Miosis. Constricted pupils.

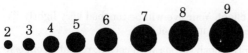

Figure 6–6. Pupil gauge chart. Size is in millimeters.

Consensual. Contraction of the pupil opposite the one being stimulated by the light.

6. Clinical alterations

    a. Decreased response of one or both eyes from lesions of the ophthalmic branch of the trigeminal nerve.

    b. Decreased response in the contact lens wearer.

J. Perform *Hirschberg's test.*

    1. Instructions to client. Look directly ahead as I shine a light into your eyes. Keep both eyes open. The light in the examining room will be dimmed for a few minutes.

    2. Technique. Hold client's head midline. Hold a lighted penlight 12 to 24 inches (30 to 60 cm) from client's head so that the light reflects off both corneas. Penlight should be in line with the bridge of the nose as client stares straight ahead.

    3. Note reflection of the dot of light on the shiny surface of each cornea.

    4. Normal finding. Light of penlight reflects as a dot on the same spot (i.e., 9 o'clock position) in both corneas.

    5. Clinical alteration. *Amblyopia:* asymmetric position of light reflex owing to loss of muscle strength of one eye.

K. Inspect the pupil.

    1. Note shape, size° (use pupil gauge chart; Fig. 6–6), symmetry, color and equality.

    2. Normal findings. Pupils equal in size°, 3 to 6 mm, round.

    3. Clinical alterations

        a. *Anisocoria* occurring congenitally, with carotid or aortic aneurysm or increased intracranial pressure.

        b. *Mydriasis* associated with hysteria, glaucoma, blindness, darkness, or mydriatic drugs

        c. *Miosis* in response to excessive light, or miotic drugs.

L. Measure the pupillary reaction to light.

    1. Equipment. Penlight, dimmed room; client seated away from bright light.

    2. Instructions to client. A light will be shone into your eyes four times. Relax and keep your eyes open, looking straight ahead. Blink as needed.

    3. Technique. Observe pupils of both eyes and compare them with pupil gauge chart (see Fig. 6–6).

        a. Direct response. Move penlight beam inward from the lateral aspect and briefly shine into client's left eye.

        b. *Consensual* (indirect) response. Flash light once again into the same left eye, observing any pupillary constriction in the right eye.

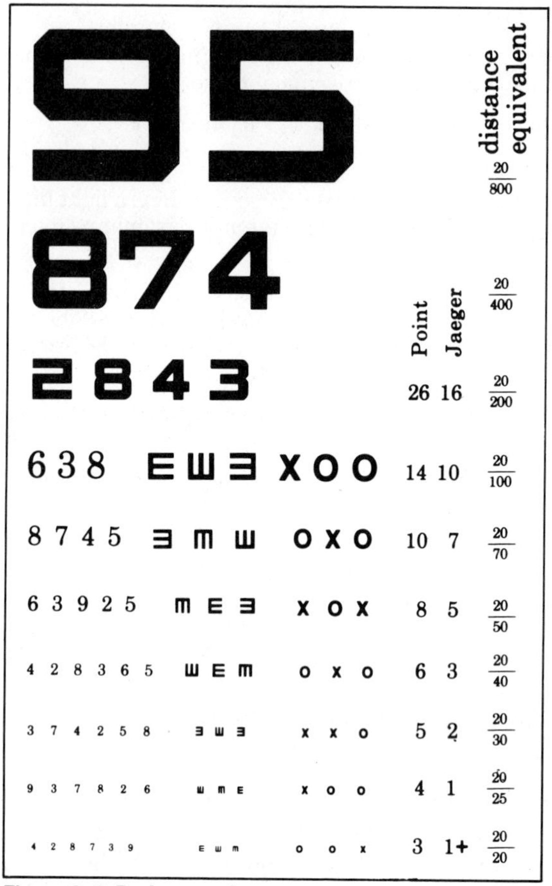

Figure 6–7. Pocket eye chart.

The client should not use his or her fingers to cover the eye because they may cause blurring of that eye from pressure. Also, the client may be tempted to peek through fingers when reading the chart.

OD: right eye   OS: left eye   OU: both eyes

The numerator is the distance in feet the client stands from the wall chart; the denominator indicates the distance at which a normal-seeing person must stand to read the chart. The higher the denominator, the worse the vision.

Presbyopia. Impairment of near vision, which develops as the client ages. Presbyopia is caused by an increase in the size of the lens owing to the continuous addition of new lens fiber through the life span, resulting in a loss in accommodation.

Myopia. Nearsightedness.

Hyperopia. Farsightedness.

  c. Repeat procedure. Place penlight in left hand and shine it into the client's right eye, first observing the right eye and then observing the left eye.

  d. Allow pupils time to relax in between times.

 4. **Note** degree of constriction of the pupil in response to direct light; simultaneous constriction of opposite pupil (speed of response may be slower in the geriatric client).

 5. **Normal findings.** Both pupils constrict in direct and consensual response to light.

 6. **Clinical alteration.** Pupils fail to react owing to retinal, optic nerve damage, or pressure in the central nervous system.

IV. Assessment of vision and ocular movements

A. Test visual acuity.

 1. **Equipment.** Small card, Snellen wall or pocket eye chart (Fig. 6–7), an E chart for children, a newspaper.

 2. **Position.** Client stands 20 feet (6 m) from wall chart or sits opposite from examiner holding pocket chart.

 3. **Instructions to client.** Read the chart from top to bottom and from right to left, beginning with the smallest line you can see clearly. Try to identify as many letters as possible. If you are unable to read, indicate the direction of the E. Wear your glasses if you are near-sighted. Cover your eye with this card, switch sides when asked to do so.° Next, read a few sentences in this newspaper.

 4. **Technique.** Have client stand 20 feet (6 m) from standard Snellen wall chart or hold the pocket version 14 inches (35 cm) from client. Encourage client to read as many letters as possible. Next, have client read a few sentences in a newspaper. Test both eyes in this same manner, with a card covering the eye not being tested.

 5. **Note** ability of the client to read the letters on each line, or to indicate the direction of the letter E. Record the eye involved° and the number next to the last line on which the client was able to identify at least half of the numbers correctly.° Also record whether the client wore glasses and was squinting or blinking.

 6. **Normal findings.** Vision 20/20 with correction. Varying degrees of *presbyopia* may develop in clients more than 40 years of age. (Having client read newspaper will detect this.)

 7. **Clinical alterations**

  a. Inability to read the smaller letters on the chart. Associated with *myopia.*

  b. Inability to read the newspaper. Associated with *hyperopia.*

Confrontation. Both the client and the examiner view the same visual fields with opposing eyes, with the examiner comparing his or her peripheral vision (which is presumed to be normal) against the client's. It is only a gross estimate.

A wiggling object is more easily seen than is a stationary object.

It is of utmost importance that the examiner's fingers be held in the midline. If the fingers are held too close to the examiner, the client will see the fingers first because they will be beyond the peripheral vision of the examiner.

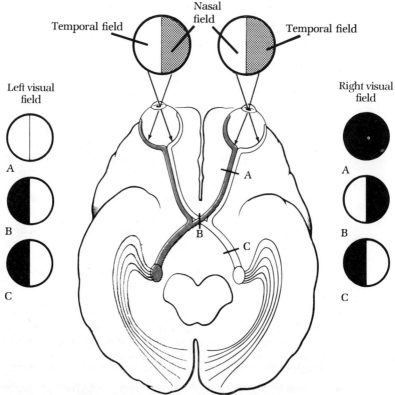

Figure 6–8. Neural pathways from the visual center of the brain to the retina. The letters represent points of lesions and resulting visual field losses. The blackened areas indicate areas of blindness: A. Blindness right eye; B. Bitemporal hemianopsia; C. Left homonymous hemianopsia.

Scotoma. Blind spots in the visual fields.

Accommodation. Constriction of the pupil as it adjusts from focusing on a distant point to a near object. The ciliary muscles constrict and the eyes converge.

B. **Test peripheral visual fields using *confrontation*.**

1. **Position.** Client and examiner directly facing each other sitting 2 feet apart.

2. **Instructions to the client.** Please remove your glasses (if applicable). Cover your right eye with this card and look directly at my right eye with your left eye. Continue to look directly at my eye and say "now" when and if you see my fingers wiggling. Do not look to the right or left.

3. **Technique.** While maintaining eye contact (opposite eyes) with the client, hold up both hands and extend both arms as if displaying an imaginary radius between yourself and the client. Wiggle one finger and then the same finger on the opposite hand,° moving toward the center, from the side of the client's head into his or her view, until the client responds. Slowly change the position of your hands around the imaginary radius, keeping your hands midway between you and the client,° moving from top to bottom. Repeat procedure, continuing until all quadrants of vision have been tested. As client covers opposite eye, repeat procedure. (With a child, it might be helpful to have the client tell examiner how many fingers are in each quadrant.)

4. **Note** ability of client to correctly identify wiggling fingers in all quadrants. Diagram any specific deficits.

5. **Normal findings.** Examiner and client should see the wiggling fingers at the same point in all quadrants.

6. **Clinical alterations** (Fig. 6–8).

    a. Decreased peripheral vision from chronic glaucoma.

    b. ***Scotoma.*** Often associated with a defect in the optic pathways.

C. **Elicit *accommodation*.**

1. **Position.** Client seated opposite examiner.

2. **Instructions to client.** Look at a distant point (a mark or object on a far wall) and then look at my finger when asked to do so.

3. **Technique.** Observe client's pupils as client looks at distant target. Quickly place finger 2 to 4 inches (5–10 cm) from client's nose and direct the client's gaze to it.

Parasympathetic fibers stimulate the oculomotor nerve, causing the pupils to constrict; sympathetic fibers cause the pupils to dilate.

Convergence. Coordinated movement of the eyes toward fixation on some near point.

Holding the penlight too low causes the lids to cover the pupils as the client looks down.

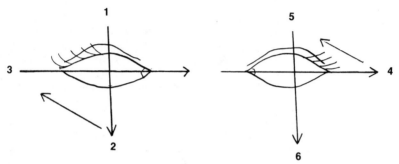

Figure 6–9. Direction of ocular movements when assessing the six cardinal fields of gaze.

Geriatric clients have difficulty focusing on objects held too close to their eyes.

The coordinated movements of the eye include abduction, adduction, elevation, depression, intorsion (toward nose), and extorsion (away from the nose).

Conjugate. Movement of the eyes together in parallel fashion in any direction.

Nystagmus. Jerking movement of the eyeball with a slow component and a rapid compensatory component in the opposite direction. The direction of the quick component is the direction of the nystagmus. Less than 40 jerks is termed slow; more than 100 is termed fast.

Ophthalmoplegia. Paralysis of eye movement. In noting the direction in which the eye will not move, the involved nerve can be identified as follows:

Oculomotor (third cranial nerve): if paralysis is down and in or up and down

Abducens (sixth cranial nerve): if paralysis is lateral

Trochlear (fourth cranial nerve): if paralysis is down and out (it is rare to find this in isolation)

The client may tilt his or her head to compensate for the paralysis.

   4. **Note** pupillary constriction of both pupils as gaze is shifted from far to near;° convergence of eyes.

   5. **Clinical alteration.** Loss of accommodation from glaucoma or injury to the retinal nerve.

D. **Measure *convergence* of eyes.**

   1. **Equipment.** Penlight.

   2. **Position.** Client seated opposite examiner.

   3. **Technique.** Hold penlight 20 inches (50 cm) from a central point on the client's face, at eye level.° Slowly and evenly direct the pen toward the bridge of the client's nose.

   4. **Note** convergence or crossing of the eyes or the point at which one or both eyes can no longer converge.

   5. **Normal findings.** Convergence of both eyes until 2 to 3 inches (5 to 7 cm) from bridge of nose.

   6. **Clinical alterations**

      a. Poor convergence in hypothyroidism.

      b. Drifting of one eye from loss of muscle function.

E. **Test extraocular movements in the six cardinal fields of gaze** (Fig. 6–9).

   1. **Instructions to client.** Look directly at me. Follow my finger with both eyes. Do not tilt or turn your head.

   2. **Technique.** Cup client's chin in nondominant hand to stabilize head. With other hand, hold up one finger 18 inches away from client's eyes.° Methodically move finger slowly and steadily up and then down over client's right eye, over to the left, across to the right, up again over left eye and down again. Keep finger within client's visual fields.

   3. **Note** the coordinated ability of both eyes to follow your finger in all six positions° and the direction and pattern of any nystagmus; lid lag.

   4. **Normal findings. *Conjugate*** movement of eyes, mild ***nystagmus*** in the elderly in the extreme lateral position.

   5. **Clinical alterations**

      a. Disconjugate gaze from weak eye muscles or ipsilateral brain lesions causing pressure on the nerves.

      b. Inability to follow examiner's finger owing to weak muscles or lesions of the brainstem or cerebellum.

      c. ***Ophthalmoplegia*** from paralysis.

      d. Nystagmus owing to various nervous system disorders.

Fundus. The posterior portion of the eye where the optic nerve and the arterioles and veins find ingress and egress in the area of the optic disc.

General principles of the ophthalmoscopic examination:

1. If the examiner needs corrective lenses, he or she should wear them to enhance visual clarity.

2. The examiner's head and ophthalmoscope should move as a single unit.

3. A diopter is a unit of measurement of the power of the lens to converge and diverge light. A black diopter is plus setting; a red diopter is minus, depending on the accommodation response and the refractive error of both the examiner and the client.

4. Move the dial from + 15 toward 0 as you progress to view objects farther within the internal structure of the eye (i.e., lens to fundus).

5. If client is nearsighted, rotate counterclockwise to the red; if client is farsighted, rotate clockwise toward the black.

6. A high refractive error will lessen the brightness of the red reflex.

7. The blood vessels increase in diameter toward the optic disc; consequently, the examiner can follow a vessel's increasing diameter to locate the optic disc.

8. The optic disc is the least light-sensitive area; the macular is the most sensitive.

9. The macular area should be examined last because it may be uncomfortable for the client.

10. The client should gaze at a distant object to enhance dilation of the pupil using accommodation; the lights in the room should be dimmed to prevent pupillary constriction in response to light.

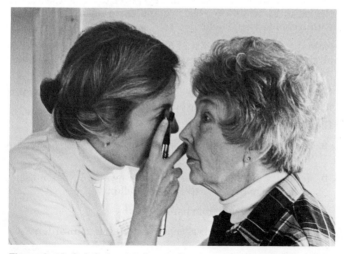

Figure 6–10. Ophthalmoscopic examination of the eye. Note that examiner's right hand and right eye face the client's right eye.

V. Ophthalmoscopic examination of the optic *fundus.* ° Inspect the internal structures of the eye.

   A. Equipment. Ophthalmoscope.

   B. Position of client. Examiner faces the lateral side of the eye being examined. Lights are dimmed.

   C. Instructions to client. A bright light will be shone through your pupil into the back of your eye. Look at fixed target on distant wall. Do not look directly at the light unless asked to do so. It may be slightly uncomfortable but it will not hurt. Blink when necessary but try not to shift your gaze from the distant target.

   D. Technique. Turn on light of the ophthalmoscope and set light beam to the large round beam for large pupils and to the small round beam for small pupils. Examine the client's right eye by holding the ophthalmoscope in your right hand, up in front of your right eye. Keep both eyes open. Stabilize client's head by placing opposite hand on top of client's head with thumb extended over right eyebrow. Place the forefinger of your right hand on the white-milled disc of the lens to easily change lens focus. Hold the ophthalmoscope 6 to 12 inches (15 to 30 cm) from the client's eye at 0 setting, approaching at a 15-degree angle, lateral to the client's direct line of vision. Direct beam on pupil to observe the red reflex. Bring the scope within 3 inches (7.5 cm) of the client's eye, rotating lens between $+10$ and -5 to bring the vitreous, then the blood vessels, into focus. Rest middle finger against client's cheek (Fig. 6–10). A 0 setting is best in the absence of refractive errors. Examine the optic disc and the physiologic cup. Last, examine the sensitive macular region by asking the client to look directly at the light for a few brief seconds. Repeat procedure for examination of the opposite eye.

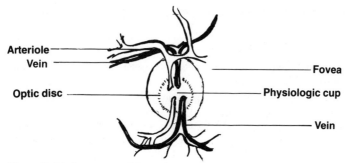

Figure 6–11. Structures of the retina.

Papilledema (choked disk). A swelling around the optic nerve associated with increased intracranial pressure.

Optic atrophy. Compression of the optic nerve causing blindness.

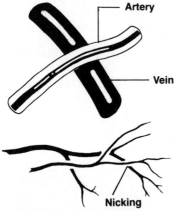

Figure 6–12. As the arteriolar wall thickens, it appears as though there is a gap between the arteriolar column of blood and the underlying vein.

E. **Note** color and opacities in the red reflex; the pattern of branching blood vessels (Fig. 6–11), color, and width of arterioles and veins, pulsating of veins, nicking of veins at arteriovenous crossing; color and margins of the physiologic cup in relation to the color and margins of the optic disc; location (in disc diameters) of any anomalies; and lesions on the retina.

F. **Normal findings.** Orange glow of red reflex; lens and vitreous body clear; bright red arteries with a strip of white light down the center, wide darker vein without a strip; a circular or vertically oval, pinkish orange to creamy yellow optic disc 1.5 mm in diameter, with the physiologic cup filling less than half of its center; the dark red, avascular macular area, located 2 to 3 disc diameters from the temporal side of the disc; with the fovea more distant in the geriatric client.

G. **Clinical alterations**

   1. Dull red or loss of reflex owing to opacities of the lens commonly caused by cataracts, especially in the client with diabetes.

   2. Blurred disc margins and full retinal veins without pulsations from *papilledema.*

   3. *Optic atrophy* associated with multiple sclerosis, glaucoma, severe papilledema, and brain tumors.

   4. Small, rounded hemorrhages seen in diabetes; flame hemorrhage in hypertension.

   5. Exudate from arteriolar microinfarctions.

   6. Arteriovenous nicking associated with atherosclerotic changes (Fig. 6–12).

VI. Chart

A. **External eye.** Eyebrows and lashes full, no exudate, edema, or scales; lids smooth without lid lag or deformity; no exaphthalmos; sclera white and clear; conjunctiva pink without injection; no tearing; iris round, flat

B. **Vision.** PERRLA, with convergence; extraocular movement intact, no nystagmus; visual fields normal by confrontation; Hirschberg's test positive; visual acuity 20/20 OU, without correction.

C. **Internal eye.** Bilateral red reflex, discs creamy pink, round with well-defined margins, 0.5 cup-disk ratio; no arteriovenous nicking; macula 2 disc diameters from optic disk; no retinal lesions, hemorrhages, or exudate.

Assessment
of the Breast

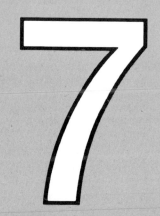

7

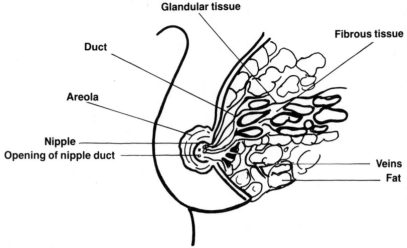

Figure 7–1. Cross section of the female breast.

Breast cancer is more prevalent in women more than 40 years of age.

Breast cancer is more common in women who either started to menstruate early or who had a late menopause.

Although breast cancer is not inherited, a woman who has female relatives—especially mother, daughter, or sister—with breast cancer is at higher risk of developing the disease.

Breast cancer is more common in women first pregnant after 30 years of age.

Self-examination of the breast should always be performed monthly after the menstrual period or, in postmenopausal women, on the same day of every month (e.g., on the client's birthday) to establish a pattern. Most cancers are initially detected by the woman herself. Although breast cancer is rare in men, breast examination should be done routinely.

Discharge from nipple may be associated with both benign and malignant diseases of the breast.

I. Clinical considerations

A. The examiner must possess a thorough understanding of the anatomy and physiology of the breast (Fig. 7–1).

B. A working knowledge of the lymphatic drainage of the breast is essential because metastasis of breast cancer cells occurs through this system.

C. The examination of the breasts includes inspection and palpation of the breasts and palpation of the lymph nodes that drain the breast.

D. Proper positioning and good lighting are key factors to inspection and palpation of the breast.

E. It is important for the examiner to acknowledge the societal association of the breast with sexuality; this makes the assessment of the breast an emotionally uncomfortable examination for many female clients.

F. Assessment of breast symmetry is essential; the client must have both breasts uncovered for comparison.

G. Ideally, the breast examination should not take place immediately before a women's menstrual period because the breast may be normally tender and engorged.

H. The breast examination provides the examiner with an excellent opportunity to demonstrate self-examination of the breast.

II. History questions relevant to the examination of the female breast

A. **Age.**°

B. **Menstruation.**° Ask questions related to the following:

   1. Age of menarche.

   2. Date of last menstrual period.

   3. Age at menopause.

C. **Family history of breast cancer.**°

D. **Childbearing.**° Ask questions related to the following:

   1. Number of children.

   2. Age when children were born.

   3. Breastfeeding pattern.

E. **Breast self-examination.**° Ask questions related to the following:

   1. When and how performed.

   2. Any findings by the client.

Note: The following questions should also be asked of male clients.

F. **Discharge from nipple.**° Ask questions related to the following:

   1. Onset, duration, amount, color, odor, consistency, and frequency.

   2. Use of medications such as birth control pills or steroids.

Breast pain (mastodynia) or lumps usually are associated with benign lesions or disorders; tenderness in the area of a lump, however, is often the first symptom of breast cancer a woman notices. Premenstrual breast pain is common in adolescents and young adults.

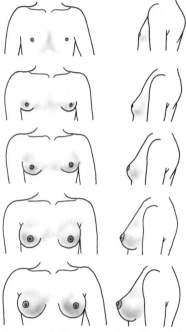

Figure 7–2. Tanner staging of female breast development.

Gynecomastia. Excessive development of the male breast.

Edema causes the hair follicles and openings to be made more pronounced, so that they resemble an "orange peel" (peau d'orange).

Veins dilate from increased vascularity in the presence of a tumor.

G. **Breast pain or lumps.**° Ask questions related to the following:

1. Onset, duration, quantity, quality, location (one or both breasts), radiation of pain, relation to menstrual cycle, and history of previous episodes.

2. Predisposing factors such as menstruation, lactation, pregnancy, or history of fibrocystic disease.

3. Associated signs and symptoms such as dimpling or retraction of skin, or discharge from the nipple.

4. Use of birth control pills.

III. **Inspection of the breast. Position** client so that she is seated upright, with arms at her side, disrobed from the waist up. Begin inspection 3 feet from the client to fully view both breasts.

A. **Compare the breasts.**

1. **Note** size, symmetry, hair pattern, location, contour, and the Tanner stage of breast development (Fig. 7–2).

2. **Normal findings.** Breasts equal bilaterally, slight asymmetry is common in adolescents; breasts extend from the third to the sixth ribs with the nipple and areola over the fourth or fifth rib; convex contour; sparse hair surrounds areola. Size of breast varies with overall body weight, genetic, and hormonal influences; flatter breasts are seen in the geriatric client.

3. **Clinical alterations**

   a. Marked asymmetry from cysts, inflammation, or tumor.

   b. *Gynecomastia,* which may occur transiently in the normal male adolescent.

B. **Assess the breast skin.**

1. **Note** color, texture, venous pattern, temperature, and the presence of edema, dimpling or retraction, and lesions.

2. **Normal findings.** Warm, smooth skin, silver striae, color lighter than exposed areas of skin.

3. **Clinical alterations**

   a. Edema and dimpling° often suggestive of breast cancer or mastitis.

   b. Inflammation often from mastitis, breast abscess, or inflammatory breast carcinoma.

   c. Retraction from a benign or malignant tumor.

   d. Dilated superficial veins from a benign or malignant tumor.°

Pigmentation varies with genetic factors and estrogen levels. The high estrogen levels of adolescence and pregnancy darken the pigment; menopause lightens it.

Supernumerary nipples. Extra nipples with a small amount of areola usually located along the "milk line."

Inversion that is long standing is considered normal.

Paget's disease. A slow-growing, intraductal carcinoma.

Observing the client in various positions causes different contractions of the pectoral muscles and suspensory ligaments, accentuating retraction. Men need only be examined sitting with arms at side.

A folded towel should be placed under the shoulder of the side being examined to allow for more even distribution of breast tissue.

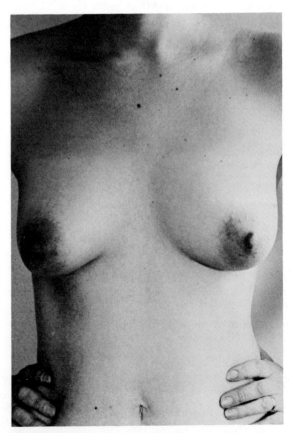

Figure 7–3. Observe breasts when client has both arms pressed firmly on hips. This position flexes the pectoral muscles.

C. **Inspect the areolae and nipples.**

1. **Note** size, shape, texture, and pigmentation° of the areolar area: direction, size, shape, pigmentation of the nipples; and the presence of any discharge or **supernumerary nipples.**

2. **Normal findings.** Symmetrically round or oval areolae, pink to dark brown, with roughened Montgomery tubercles; nipples erect, same color as areolae.

3. **Clinical alterations**

   a. Inversion often associated with breast cancer.°

   b. Excoriation often associated with **Paget's disease.**

D. Observe breasts as described in **A, B,** and **C** when the client is in the following positions:°

1. Sitting with both arms raised over head.

2. Sitting with both arms pressed firmly on hips, flexing pectoral muscles (Fig. 7–3).

3. Sitting, leaning forward with arms outstretched, allowing breasts to hang freely.

4. Supine with arm above head, on the side being examined.°

Breast self-examination should be performed in front of a mirror at home.

Lubrication facilitates the sliding of the fingerpads over the breast. The client can use this same technique in the bath or shower.

Charting location (quadrant) and extent of anomalies of the breasts on a diagram is the most precise way to record them. The diagram should include horizontal and vertical lines intersecting at the nipple, dividing the breast into four quadrants.

Fibroadenomas. Generalized, lumpy, tender breasts occurring in nulliparous women between the ages of 30 and 50.

Breast cancer. Solitary, nontender breast mass fixed to the pectoral muscles, with retraction and dimpling of the skin, flattening of the nipple, and a clear discharge from a single duct.

Chronic mastitis. Tender, multiple nodules with no retraction or dimpling. Nodules and tenderness increase prior to menstruation.

The areola is the more common site for breast carcinoma in men, so particular attention should be made here when examining the male breast.

Nipple discharge from multiple ducts is suggestive of benign disease of the breast; discharge from a single duct is suggestive of cancer.

Stimulation of the nipple during palpation will cause it to become erect and puckered.

IV. Palpation of the breast. Position client so that she is sitting with both arms at her sides.

   A. Palpate the four quadrants of the breast.

      1. **Instructions to client.** Observe how your breast is being examined so that you can use this technique at home.° Describe any tenderness.

      2. **Technique.** Examiner should lubricate his or her fingers with lotion or soap and warm water.° Gently palpate the breast with the pads of the four fingers. Starting at the 12 o'clock position on the upper aspect of the breast, rotate fingerpads in imaginary concentric circles, rotating toward the center of the breast, areola, and nipple. Do not lift fingers from the breast. In large-breasted women, use bimanual palpation, compressing breast between hands. Next, palpate the breast with client supine, with arm above head on the side being examined. Repeat for other breast. Chart any anomalies.°

      3. **Note** temperature; size, location, degree of fixation; consistency of any masses; and breast tenderness.

      4. **Normal findings.** Breast warm, smooth, elastic; no masses or discharge; coarser and more nodular in the geriatric client.

      5. **Clinical alterations**

         a. Nontender, mobile, well-delineated nodules associated with *fibroadenomas.*

         b. Nontender, immobile, or fixed nodule suggestive of *breast cancer.*

         c. Tender, multiple nodes in one or both breasts from *chronic mastitis.*

   B. Palpate nipple and areola.°

      1. **Technique.** Gently compress nipple between index finger and thumb. Repeat for other nipple. Specimens of any discharge should be sent to a laboratory for cytologic examination.

      2. **Note** the amount, color, odor, and number of ducts any fluid is ejected from;° shape and consistency of nipple.

      3. **Normal findings.** No discharge, except during lactation; nipple erect.°

      4. **Clinical alterations**

         a. Unilateral, serous, or serosanguinous discharge suggestive of introductal pappillomas.

         b. Clear, yellowish fluid associated with chronic mastitis.

         c. Sanguinous or dark red discharge associated with Paget's disease.

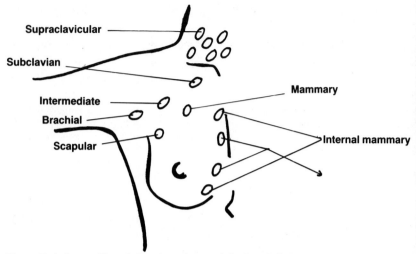

Figure 7–4. Areas of lymph flow in and around the female breast.

C. Palpate lymph nodes (Fig. 7–4).

1. **Technique.** Using the same rotating motion, gently palpate the clavicular area. Face the patient, abduct her right arm with your right hand and place your left hand against the chest wall, high into the axilla. Rotate your hand, using gentle pressure to palpate the subscapular, central, pectoral, and lateral axillary nodes. Repeat for opposite axilla. Repeat with client supine with arm over her head.

2. **Note** location (which quadrant), size (in centimeters), shape, consistency, mobility, and tenderness.

3. **Normal findings.** None.

4. **Clinical alterations**

   a. Nontender, hard enlarged lymph nodes indicative of metastatic breast cancer.

   b. Lymphadenitis from an infection of the client's arm.

V. Chart. Breasts symmetric, normal contour, no dimpling, retraction, or erythema; nipples erect, no discharge; areola pink; firm, smooth, elastic breasts; no masses or palpable lymph nodes.

Assessment
of the Thorax
and Lungs

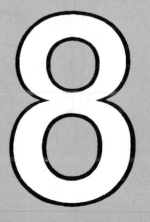

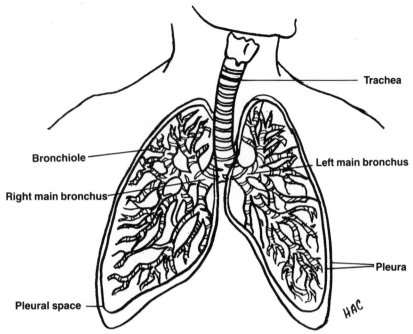

Figure 8–1. Anatomy of the lungs.

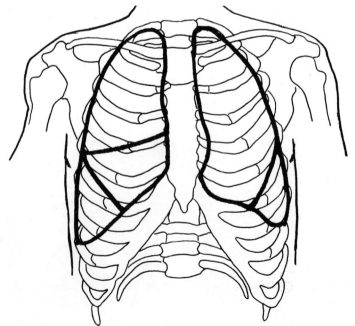

Figure 8–2. Lungs under the bones of the thorax.

I. Clinical considerations

A. The examiner must possess a thorough understanding of the anatomy and physiology of the thorax and lungs (Figs. 8–1, 8–2).

B. The examination of the thorax and lungs includes inspection and palpation of the thorax and percussion and auscultation of the lungs.

C. The examiner must observe the client closely throughout the examination to detect any signs of lightheadedness from hyperventilation.

D. The posterior thorax and lungs are examined first while the client is sitting; the lateral and anterior aspects are next examined while the client is supine.

E. Respiratory excursion, diaphragmatic excursion, and fremitus are usually best assessed using the posterior approach; percussion and auscultation must also include the anterior thorax and lungs in order to assess the right middle lobe.

F. The base of the fingers is more sensitive to vibratory changes than the fingertips when assessing fremitus.

G. Location of any clinical alterations should be described in centimeters from the midsternal line and in interspaces. The midclavicular lines are not exact.

H. Assessment of the lungs and thorax is especially important in the geriatric client and in the child because of the many respiratory diseases that affect these two groups.

I. Assessment of symmetry involves using the side-to-side comparison as a norm for that particular client.

Cough. A noisy, forceful blast of air expelled from the lungs, out the mouth and nose. It is the result of contraction of the abdominal and expiratory muscles. It is the most common respiratory symptom. Coughing is a protective mechanism that may be stimulated by internal factors such as an allergic or an inflammatory resonse or external irritants such as inhaling smoke or dust. A paroxysmal cough is suggestive of bronchial obstruction. A cough may be caused by cardiac diseases such as congestive heart failure or mitral valve disease. An unproductive cough does not raise sputum; a productive cough raises sputum and is usually longer in duration.

Shortness of breath (dyspnea). Uncomfortable or difficult breathing. Exertional dyspnea may be due to restrictive causes within the rib cage or obstructive causes owing to airway resistance. Clients with restrictive dyspnea are comfortable at rest but become short of breath on exertion. Clients with obstructive disease are short of breath with labored breathing even at rest. With orthopnea associated with congestive heart failure, the client needs to sit up to breathe comfortably. Orthopnea is often described in terms of number of pillows needed to sleep without dyspnea (e.g., two-pillow orthopnea).

Hemoptysis. Spitting or coughing up blood as a result of bleeding from the capillaries or major large blood vessels of the respiratory tract. Inflammatory causes, such as bronchitis or an upper respiratory tract infection, account for most cases of hemoptysis. Bronchogenic cancer must be suspected in heavy smokers more than 40 years of age. Hemoptysis associated with chest pain is indicative of pulmonary infarction. Any bright red blood expectorated in excess of 2 teaspoons may signal frank hemorrhage. Causes of hemoptysis other than pulmonary must also be explored (i.e., bleeding esophageal varices).

II. Relevant history questions

A. *Cough.* Ask questions related to the following:

1. Onset, duration, exposure to pollutants, character (dry, hacking, coarse), pattern (time of day), and history of recent upper respiratory tract infections, previous episodes, or family allergies.

2. Predisposing factors such as stress, recent upper respiratory tract infection, tobacco smoking, inhalation of toxic gases, or a known lung disorder.

3. Associated signs and symptoms such as chest pain, sputum production (character), shortness of breath, orthopnea (number of pillows), or fever.

4. Use of therapeutic modalities such as analgesics, cough medicine, or vaporizer.

B. *Shortness of breath.* Ask questions related to the following:

1. Onset, pattern (how many stairs or blocks), character, duration, and history of previous episodes or cardiopulmonary disease.

2. Predisposing factors such as stress, recent upper respiratory tract infection, excessive tobacco use, thoracic deformity, or exertion.

3. Associated signs and symptoms such as cough, orthopnea (number of pillows), diaphoresis, increased or decreased respirations.

C. *Hemoptysis.* Ask questions related to the following:

1. Onset, duration, amount (in teaspoons), pattern, character (color), and history of previous episodes or trauma.

2. Predisposing factors such as previously diagnosed respiratory disease, excessive alcohol and tobacco use, or recent upper respiratory tract infection.

3. Associated signs and symptoms such as chest pain, cough, fever, or shortness of breath.

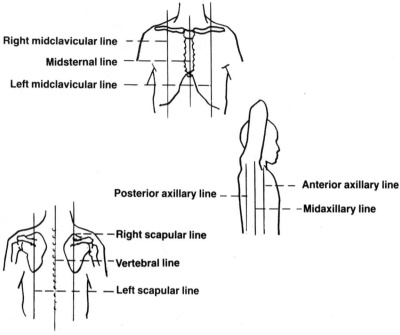

Figure 8–3. Imaginary lines of the chest.

Muscles of respiration relax during expiration and the thorax springs back into shape.

Accessory muscles. Additional muscles needed for breathing during times of increased respiratory effort. They are the pectoral, scalene, sternocleidomastoid, and trapezius muscles.

Hyperpnea. Abnormally deep and rapid breathing exceeding 20 respirations per minute.

Bradypnea. Abnormally slow breathing less than 12 respirations per minute.

Kussmaul's respirations (air hunger). Very deep, gasping respirations.

Cheyne-Stokes respirations. Abnormal periods of deep breathing alternating with periods of apnea.

III. Inspection of the thorax. Position client so that he or she is sitting upright, undressed to the waist, and draped appropriately. Begin inspection 3 feet from the client to view the entire thorax, visualizing the lungs beneath the surface landmarks (Fig. 8–3).

A. **Assess respiratory pattern.**°

    1. **Note** rate, depth, and rhythm of inspiration and expiration, the presence of any audible sounds, posture and comfort, use of **accessory muscles,** and bulging or retraction of interspaces.

    2. **Normal findings.** Quiet respirations, 1 : 4 ratio of respiratory rate to heart rate, 12 to 20 respirations per minute in adults, 20 to 24 in children; symmetric rise and fall of chest without discomfort; use of diaphragm in men and children, ribs in women; no use of accessory muscles of respiration or bulging or retraction of interspaces.

    3. **Clinical alterations**

        a. *Hyperpnea* often from exercise, anxiety, or fever.

        b. *Bradypnea* often from diabetic coma or increased intracranial pressure.

        c. *Kussmaul's respirations* often associated with metabolic acidosis.

        d. *Cheyne-Stokes respirations* often from heart failure, anemia, or brain damage.

        e. Use of accessory muscles of respiration owing to respiratory distress with increased respiratory effort.

        f. Bulging of interspaces from emphysema.

        g. Sighing respirations associated with anxiety and hyperventilation.

B. **Compare the anterior posterior diameter to the lateral diameter.**

    1. **Note** the ratio of the anterior or the posterior view to the lateral view.

    2. **Normal findings.** The anterior posterior diameter is less than the lateral diameter; 1 : 2 or 5 : 7.

    3. **Clinical alteration.** Increase in the diameter owing to a barrel chest, often associated with emphysema.

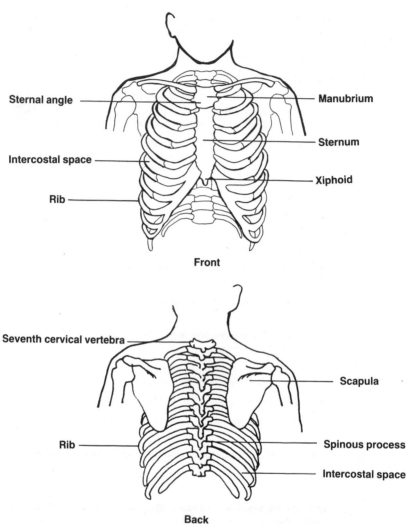

Figure 8–4. Skeletal structures of the thorax.

An asymetric chest is the result of either abnormal bony structures or abnormal contents within the thorax.

Kyphosis (humpback). Accentuated posterior convex curvature of the thoracic spine.

Lordosis (swayback). Accentuated anterior convex curvature of the lumbar spine.

Scoliosis. Lateral curvature of the thoracic spine.

C. **Assess the configuration of the skeletal structures of the thorax°** (Fig. 8–4).

1. **Note** the curvature of the spine, slope of the ribs, costal angle, and angle and symmetry of the scapulae.

2. **Normal findings.** Midline and spine straight, scapulae even, costal angle less than 90 degrees in adults and 45 degrees in children, mild kyphosis in the geriatric client.

3. **Clinical alterations**

   a. Increased costal angle often associated with emphysema.

   b. Pectus carinatum (pigeon chest) associated with rickets.

   c. Pectus excavatum (funnel chest) owing to pulmonary emphysema or senile kyphosis.

   d. *Kyphosis* associated with ankylosing spondylitis, Paget's disease, acromegaly, or senile osteoporosis.

   e. *Lordosis* associated with weakness of back muscles, obesity, or ankylosis of hips.

   f. *Scoliosis* often congenitally acquired; first noted in the school-age child.

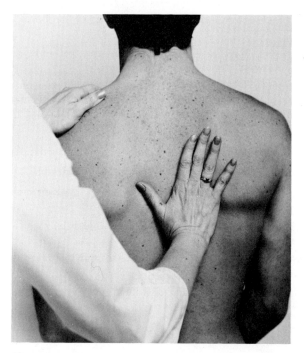

Figure 8–5. Palpation of the back using a circular motion.

Rachitic rosary. Bulging of the costochondral junctions owing to rickets.

Crepitations (subcutaneous emphysema). Audible crackling of small air pockets in the subcutaneous tissue.

IV. **Palpation of the thorax. Position** client so that he or she is seated upright for palpation of the posterior thorax and supine for palpation of the anterior and lateral thorax.

    A. **Palpate skin and underlying structures.**

        1. **Instructions to client.** Describe any tenderness.

        2. **Technique.** Place fingerpads on top of shoulders. Using a gentle, circular motion, systematically progress across and downward over the entire rib cage (Fig. 8–5). Palpate sternal notch.

        3. **Note** temperature, texture, moisture, and tenderness of the skin; masses; tenderness of the muscles or costochondral junctions; pulsations of the aorta and position of the trachea in the sternal notch.

        4. **Normal findings.** Warm, moist, smooth skin; no tenderness; mild pulsations in sternal notch; trachea midline.

        5. **Clinical alterations**

            a. Tenderness from pleurisy, myositis, or *rachitic rosary.*

            b. *Crepitations* owing to leaking of air from a pneumothorax.

Respiratory excursion. Measurement of thoracic expansion during inspiration as compared to expiration. The thumbs will not easily slide if too much pressure is applied.

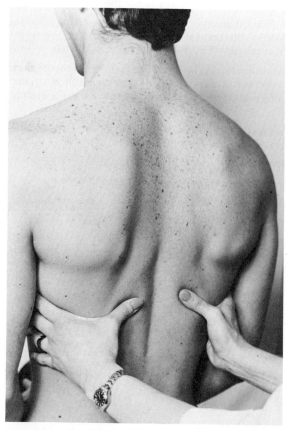

Figure 8–6. Assessment of respiratory excursion using the posterior approach. Note thumbs at the level of T-10.

Fremitus. Low-pitched, palpable vibrations felt through the chest wall when the client speaks. Noting the amount and pitch of the vibrations enables the examiner to assess the adequate flow of air through the bronchi and alveoli as it is transmitted to the chest wall.

B. **Measure *respiratory excursion*.**

   1. **Instructions to client.** Inhale and exhale deeply through open mouth when asked to do so.

   2. **Technique.** Lightly place thumbs on either side of the tenth thoracic vertebrae (T-10) in the midline and extend fingers laterally around ribs (Fig. 8–6). As client takes a deep breath, allow hands to slide with inspiration and expiration.

   3. **Note** symmetry and movement of rib cage as lungs expand.

   4. **Normal findings.** Smooth movement, equal expansion with thumbs moving symmetrically apart during inspiration and sliding back together during expiration; decreased chest expansion in women and in the geriatric client.

   5. **Clinical alterations**

     a. Decreased expansion of the thorax often associated with pain, ankylosing spondylitis, or pulmonary fibrosis.

     b. Asymmetry of expansion owing to impaired function of one lung from pneumonia or fractured ribs.

C. **Assess vibratory *fremitus*.**

   1. **Instructions to client.** Say "ninety-nine" every time you feel my palm touch your back. Always use the same pitch and intensity in your voice when speaking. Describe any dizziness.

Principles of palpating for fremitus:

1. Low-pitched sounds are better felt than auscultated.

2. Anything that increases the distance from the skin surface to the lungs (fat, thick muscle) will decrease fremitus.

3. If unable to adequately assess fremitus, instruct the client to speak louder and deeper.

4. Respiratory conditions that increase fremitus also increase breath sounds and vice versa.

5. A liquid or elastic solid medium increases fremitus; a nonelastic solid medium decreases fremitus.

6. The same hand should be used to palpate fremitus at all places because vibratory sensation may vary between hands.

7. Fremitus is not accurately palpated over bony areas.

8. Repeated exhaling of words may cause the client to hyperventilate.

9. The examiner's hand on the client's shoulder provides support to the client and leverage for the examiner.

10. Fremitus will normally decrease from side to side as the examiner proceeds down the thorax.

Tracheal bifurcation. Area where trachea divides into left and right main bronchi. It is posteriorly found at the level of the fourth thoracic vertebrae (T-4); anteriorly at the angle of Louis.

2. **Technique.**° Place nondominant hand on client's shoulder. Place palmar base of fingers of dominant hand opposite the seventh cervical vertibrae posteriorly. Hold fingertips up so as not to dampen vibrations. Systematically progress downward at 5-cm intervals. Do not palpate over bony areas. Palpate corresponding areas of lung fields.

3. **Note** the intensity of vibrations in corresponding areas; any dizziness of the client.

4. **Normal findings.** Equal vibrations bilaterally and a symmetric decrease toward the base. Fremitus is more intense in children than in adults because of their thin chest walls; fremitus may be decreased in women because of their higher-pitched voices. Fremitus increases in intensity over the area of the ***tracheal bifurcation.***

5. **Clinical alterations**

   a. Increased fremitus from pulmonary fibrosis, tumor, or lung consolidation.

   b. Decreased fremitus from fluid or air in the pleural space, bronchial obstruction, or a weak voice.

The drooping of the shoulders separates the scapulae and increases access to lung fields.

Percussion and auscultation of the anterior lungs should be assessed, with client supine, at the completion of the examination of the posterior thorax and lungs.

Mediate percussion. Striking an object on top of the area to be examined to assess vibration of underlying lung (to a depth of 5–7 cm) to establish the presence of air, fluid, or solid. A change in percussion note is best assessed when tapping from areas of resonance to dull.

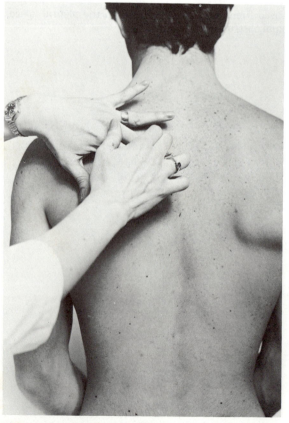

Figure 8–7. Percussion of the lung.

V. **Percussion of the lungs. Position** client so that he or she is upright with shoulders slightly drooped, head bent forward, and arms folded at the waist.° Arms should be elevated with hands on head as lateral walls are percussed. The client should lie supine for anterior percussion with examiner on right.° **Instruct** client to breathe in and out through open mouth. Women should displace their breasts as necessary.

A. **Assess relative densities of lung tissue.**

1. **Technique.** *Mediate percussion.* Beginning at the apices, place distal phalanx of nondominant hand (pleximeter) horizontally against the area to be percussed. Hold the other fingers off the skin surface. With the tip of the index finger of the dominant hand, lightly but firmly strike the first joint using rapid wrist movement. Quickly withdraw. Movement must not involve the shoulder or elbow. Tap each area twice to register tone. Proceed downward from apices, percussing each intercostal space and comparing each interspace sequentially with the percussion note from the contralateral region (Fig. 8–7).

Recognition of the various percussion notes cannot be categorized but can be gained only through repeated exposure to their characteristics. Practice on your own body to develop proficiency in recognizing the following sounds:

Tympany: over gastric air bubble or bowel

Resonance: over lungs

Dull: over the heart or liver

Flat: over thick muscle

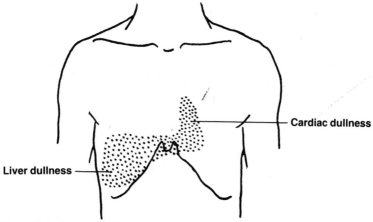

Figure 8–8. Areas of dullness of the anterior thorax.

2. **Note** percussion note in all areas.°

3. **Normal findings**

   a. **Anterior lungs.** Percussion note resonant and equal bilaterally; note slightly more resonant in upper margins of the lungs. Dull areas are found over liver (fourth to sixth interspaces in the midclavicular line) and heart (third to fifth interspaces to the left of the sternum) (Fig. 8–8).

   b. **Posterior lungs.** Percussion note resonant and equal bilaterally. Slight decrease in resonance over scapular muscles. Zone of resonance of lung bases ends in the vicinity of the ninth rib.

   c. **Apices.** Band of resonance 4 to 6 cm over each shoulder at Krönig's isthmus.

   d. Percussion note may be hyperresonant in children because of the thinness of their chest wall.

4. **Clinical alterations**

   a. Hyperresonance from increased amounts of air in the lung commonly associated with emphysema.

   b. Dullness over fluid-filled areas commonly associated with pneumonia or atelectasis.

Diaphragmatic excursion. Comparison of the level of the diaphragm on full inspiration and on full expiration. It measures the capacity of the lungs to expand and the proper functioning of the diaphragm.

On inspiration the dome-shaped diaphragm moves downward; on expiration it passively springs back.

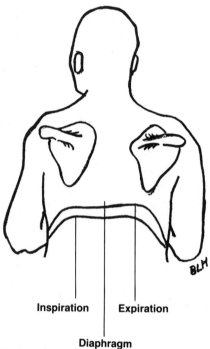

Inspiration   **Expiration**

Diaphragm

Figure 8–9. Normal diaphragmatic excursion between full inspiration and full expiration.

B. Measure *diaphragmatic excursion* (Fig. 8–9).

    1. **Equipment.** Centimeter ruler, skin-marking pencil.

    2. **Instructions to client.** Breathe in and out normally; then exhale forcibly and hold your breath for a few seconds.° Describe any dizziness.

    3. **Technique.** Mediate percussion. As client holds breath on full expiration, begin below the scapula and quickly percuss down the scapular line in each interspace. Mark area where percussion note changes from resonant (lung) to dull (muscle of the diaphragm). Instruct client to breathe normally. Next, as client holds breath on full inspiration, percuss area just marked. The note should now be resonant. Continue down the scapular line, again noting area where percussion note changes from resonant to dull. Mark area and measure the difference between the two marks in centimeters. Repeat procedure on the opposite side.

    4. **Note** any lowering of the change in percussion note on full inspiration. Compare the levels on corresponding sides. Note any dizziness of the client.

    5. **Normal findings.** Difference between full expiration and full inspiration is 3 to 6 cm in men, 3 cm in women and in the geriatric client. Full inspiration is at the level of the twelfth thoracic vertebrae (T-12); full expiration is at the level of T-10. The level may be slightly higher on the right owing to liver dullness.

    6. **Clinical alterations**

        a. Decrease or no change in the level of excursion commonly from emphysema, paralysis of the phrenic nerve, or bronchitis.

        b. Increased excursion with atelectasis or pleural effusion.

        c. Upward displacement of the diaphragm owing to obesity or pregnancy.

General considerations when using the stethoscope:

1. The diaphragm of the stethoscope picks up the higher-pitched sounds; the bell, the lower.

2. The diaphragm should be firmly pressed against the skin; the bell lightly applied so as not to create a tight seal.

3. Breathing on the tubing and rubbing the tubes against each other may create artifact and cause the examiner to misinterpret breath sounds.

4. Use the largest earpieces necessary to snugly fit into the auditory meatus.

5. Tubing should be thick and no more than 12 inches (30 cm) long.

6. Chest hair should be moistened with water.

7. A child should be allowed to handle the stethoscope because it may be frightening to him or her.

8. The chest piece should be warmed.

Table 8–1. Normal breath sounds

Breath sound	Location	Pitch	Duration	Quality
Vesicular	Over peripheral alveoli	Low	I > e	Soft rustling
Bronchovesicular	Over area around bronchial bifurcation	Moderate	I = E	Muffled blowing
Bronchial	Over trachea	High	E > i	Harsh, tubular

I(i) = inspiration; E (e) = expiration.

Adventitious sounds. Abnormal breath sounds. Descriptions of selected types follow:

Rales. Discontinuous, inspiratory sounds that are wet and crackling usually from fluid in the airways. If rales can be eliminated with coughing, they have little clinical significance.

Rhonchi. Continuous, expiratory sounds:

1. Sibilant: high-pitched whistling sounds owing to constriction of smooth muscle or fluid in the smaller airways

2. Sonorous: low-pitched, harsh, snoring sounds owing to fluid in or constriction of the larger airways

Pleural friction rub. Graty, leathery squeak owing to inflammation of the pleura causing it to lose its lubrication (sometimes called *dry wheeze*).

VI. Auscultation of the lungs. Necessary **equipment** is a stethoscope° with bell and diaphragm; a smaller diaphragm is used for children. **Instruct** client to take slow, deep breaths through open mouth and not to breathe too forcibly or dizziness may occur. **Position** client as in **V.** Make sure a child does not turn his or her head as this compresses the delicate bronchi and causes decreased breath sounds.

A. Assess breath sounds.

1. **Technique.** Firmly place diaphragm of the stethoscope on client's back. Auscultate from apex to base at 5-cm intervals, moving from side to side (as with percussion). Listen to at least one cycle of inspiration and expiration in each area. Compare sounds heard from corresponding lung fields. To auscultate anteriorly, begin at apices and again progress downward.

2. **Note** the presence of breath sounds or abnormal sounds.

3. **Normal findings.** Normal breath sounds in the areas where they are supposed to be (Table 8–1). Breath sounds will be harsher in thin adults and children.

    a. *Vesicular* breath sounds heard over the lung periphery.

    b. *Bronchovesicular* sounds heard in the area around the bifurcation of the trachea.

    c. *Bronchial* sounds heard over the larynx and cervical trachea.

4. **Clinical alterations**

    a. Decreased breath sounds owing to a decrease in the flow of air often caused by bronchial obstruction, muscular weakness, or shallow breathing.

    b. Decreased breath sounds from chronic obstructive pulmonary disease or lung consolidation.

    c. Any normal breath sounds in an area where they are not normally heard.

    d. *Adventitious sounds*

        (1) *Rales* often from congestive heart failure.

        (2) *Rhonchi* often associated with asthma.

        (3) *Pleural friction rub* from pleurisy.

Table 8–2. Anomalies of fremitus, percussion, and breath sounds in relation to common respiratory disorders

Normal or disorder	Percussion note	Fremitus	Breath sound	Adventitious sound
Normal	Resonant	+	Vesicular	None
Consolidation	Dull	↑	Bronchial	Rales
Bronchitis	Resonant	+	+	Rhonchi
Emphysema	Hyperresonant	↓	↓ Vesicular	Medium rales
Pneumothorax	Hyperresonant	↓	↓	None
Atelectasis	Dull	↓ −	↓ −	None

− = absent; + = present; ↑ = increased; ↓ = decreased.

Fluid transmits sound better than air, transmitting voice sounds more distinctly.

Note: If anomalies of fremitus, percussion, and/or breath sounds are found, proceed to B (Table 8–2). **If not, proceed to VII.**

B. **Test for bronchophony.**

1. **Instructions to client.** Say "ninety-nine" when the stethoscope is placed on your chest.

2. **Technique.** Auscultate over area of suspected anomaly.

3. **Note** quality of sound heard through the stethoscope.

4. **Normal findings.** Muffled sound exaggerated over trachea and right upper lobe.

5. **Clinical alteration.** Increase in loudness and clarity of spoken word owing to mucous- or fluid-filled alveoli.°

C. **Elicit whispered pectoriloquy.**

1. **Instructions to client.** Say "one, two, three" as the stethoscope is placed on your chest.

2. **Technique.** Auscultate over area of suspected anomaly.

3. **Note** sound heard through the stethoscope.

4. **Normal finding.** Muffled sound.

5. **Clinical alteration.** Increase in loudness and clarity of spoken word from consolidation.

D. **Assess egophony.**

1. **Instructions to client.** Say "e-e-e-e-e-e" when the stethoscope is placed on your chest.

2. **Technique.** Auscultate over area of suspected anomaly. Compare with normal area.

3. **Note** quality of sound heard through the stethoscope.

4. **Normal finding.** Muffled sound.

5. **Clinical alteration.** Increase in pitch with a nasal "a" sound like the bleating of a goat often heard over a pleural effusion.

VII. **Chart.** Respirations 14, smooth and even without effort; AP diameter 1 : 2; respiratory excursion equal bilaterally; spine straight, costal angle 90 degrees; good muscle development, diaphragmatic breathing, negative use of accessory muscles; skin warm and moist; no tenderness, pulsations, or crepitations; vibratory fremitus present and equal bilaterally; diaphragmatic excursion 3 cm and equal bilaterally; lungs resonant, normovesicular breath sounds, no rales, rhonchi, or rubs.

Assessment of the Heart and Peripheral Vascular System

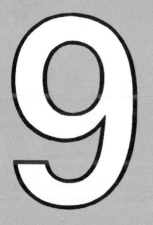

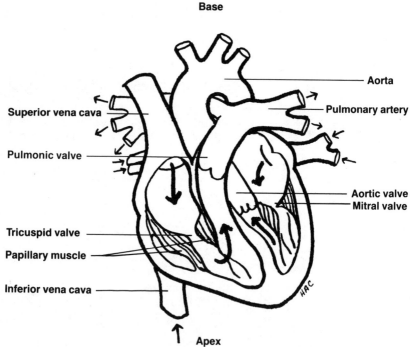

Figure 9–1. Flow of blood through the heart. Arrows indicate direction of blood flow.

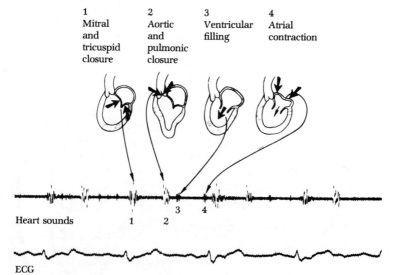

Figure 9–2. Origin of heart sounds with correlation to the phonocardiogram and electrocardiogram.

I. Clinical considerations

A. The examiner must possess a thorough understanding of the anatomy and physiology of the heart (Fig. 9–1).

B. The examination of the heart includes inspection and palpation of the precordium, percussion of cardiac borders, and auscultation of heart and vascular sounds.

C. The examination of the peripheral vascular system includes assessment of blood pressure, inspection and palpation of the peripheral pulses and lymph nodes, and measurement of the jugular venous pressure.

D. The heart is first assessed with the client supine and then sitting upright. The left lateral decubitus position may be used to clarify abnormal findings.

E. Clinical alterations should be described in terms of centimeters from the midsternal line and in interspaces.

F. To accurately auscultate the heart, the examiner must thoroughly understand the relationship of heart sounds to the mechanical events of the heart (Fig. 9–2).

G. Assessment of cardiovascular function in the child additionally includes observation of health status including color, growth and development, nutritional state, and energy level.

H. The geriatric population has a higher incidence of cardiovascular disease than young adults or children.

I. Clients are apprehensive when the heart and peripheral vascular system are examined because they fear that they have a cardiovascular disease.

J. The broader base of the heart is located above the rounder apex. Therefore, the base of the heart is at the top and the apex of the heart is located at the bottom of the chest.

Chest pain rarely presents with physical signs so obtaining an accurate history is essential. Pain intensified by thoracic movement is often designated as respiratory pain. The ribs, cartilages, muscles, nerves, and pleurae must be carefully assessed. The client with deep pain or pressure behind the sternum readily seeks medical care because of fear of cardiac disease. Angina pectoris is deep, steady pain that is usually brought on with exertion and is relieved in 1 to 10 minutes by rest and nitroglycerine. In contrast, an acute myocardial infarction lasts more than 20 minutes and is unrelieved by nitroglycerine. The client becomes hypotensive. An attack of acute pericarditis is usually accompanied by fever. A client with a dissecting aortic aneurysm maintains blood pressure, with a progressive loss of affected pulses.

Palpitation. Unusually rapid or irregular heart beat. A palpitation is a conscious, frightening sensation clients usually describe as "pounding" or "flopping" of the heart. It is often caused by minor disturbances such as exercise, excessive nicotine or caffeine, anxiety, or simply an increased awareness of one's own heart beat. Other causes are high cardiac output (i.e., hyperthyroidism), pressure on the heart (i.e., tumor), and drugs (i.e., epinephrine).

Edema. Local or generalized accumulation of excessive fluid in the interstitial tissue. Edema may be due to tissue inflammation, fluid retention, prolonged sitting or standing, incompetent leg veins, obstruction of the vena cava, lymphedema, cirrhosis, or congestive heart failure. Edema caused by heart failure often appears in the lower extremities and may be accompanied by dyspnea.

II. Relevant history questions

A. Chest pain.° Ask questions related to the following:

1. Onset, location, duration, quality, quantity, region, radiation, timing, and history of cardiopulmonary disease and previous episodes.

2. Predisposing factors such as anxiety, a large meal, recent upper respiratory tract infection, trauma to the chest, muscle strain, exertion, hyperlipidemia, or hyptertension.

3. Associated signs and symptoms such as cough, shortness of breath, tenderness over muscles and bones, palpitations, edema, nausea and vomiting, fatigue, or syncope.

4. Use of therapeutic modalities such as analgesics, nitroglycerine, or rest.

B. *Palpitation.* Ask questions related to the following:

1. Onset, duration, character, pattern, frequency, regularity, and history of previous episodes.

2. Predisposing factors such as stress, strenuous exercise, excessive coffee, tea, or alcohol intake, thyrotoxicosis, drug use, or a known cardiac disorder.

3. Associated signs and symptoms such as chest pain or a twinge in the chest, shortness of breath, cough, anxiety, fatigue, or syncope.

C. Shortness of breath. See Chapter 8, **II. B.**

D. *Edema.* Ask questions related to the following:

1. Onset, duration, extent (localized or generalized), pitting, distribution, recent weight gain, and history of previous episodes or cardiopulmonary disease.

2. Predisposing factors such as peripheral vascular disease, restrictive clothing, bed rest, obesity, or known kidney or cardiac disease, particularly congestive heart failure.

3. Associated signs and symptoms such as orthopnea (number of pillows), shortness of breath, chest pain, leg pain, or lymphadenopathy.

The examiner should always stand to the right of the client whether or not he or she is right-handed.

Tangential lighting. Light shining from a single light source from the client's left, creating shadows on his or her chest to detect any movement of the precordium. The client is lying between the examiner and the light source.

Precordium. The anterior surface of the chest that lies closest to the heart. The right ventricle dominates the anterior surface of the heart; the left ventricle lies posteriorly.

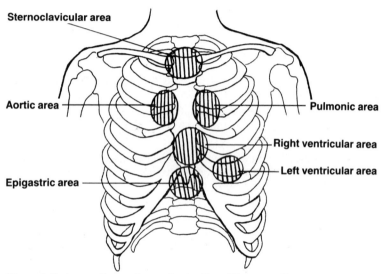

Figure 9–3. Areas of inspection and palpation of the precordium.

Left ventricular hypertrophy. Enlargement of the left ventricle associated with left-side congestive heart failure.

Right ventricular hypertrophy. Enlargement of the right ventricle associated with right-side congestive heart failure and pulmonary hypertension.

Precordial bulge. An outward protrusion of the thorax over the precordium.

III. **Inspection of the heart. Position** client so that he or she is supine, undressed to the waist. Examiner is on the client's right.° Provide *tangential lighting.* Instruct client to breathe normally. Ask large-breasted women to hold the left breast up and to the left.

   A. **Assess the shape of the thorax.** See Chapter 8, **III. C.**

   B. Inspect the *precordium* for pulsations.

   1. **Technique.** Critically inspect the following areas systematically (Fig. 9–3):

      a. **Sternoclavicular area.** Space surrounding the junction of the sternum and the clavicle.

      b. **Aortic area.** Second and third interspaces to the right of the sternum.

      c. **Pulmonic area.** Second and third interspaces to the left of the sternum.

      d. **Right ventricular area.** Lower half of the sternum, including the third and fourth interspaces to the left of the sternum.

      e. **Left ventricular area.** At the cardiac apex.

      f. **Epigastric area.** Area around the xiphoid process.

   2. **Note** location, diameter, duration, and regularity of any visible pulsations; bulging or retraction of interspaces.

   3. **Normal findings.** Slight pulsations may be seen in children and thin adults.

   4. **Clinical alterations**

      a. Increased pulsations in the sternoclavicular area owing to an aneurysm.

      b. Increased pulsations in apical area often caused by *left ventricular hypertrophy.*

      c. Increased pulsations medial to the apex in the third, fourth, or fifth interspace often caused by *right ventricular hypertrophy.*

      d. *Precordial bulge* seen in children with congenital heart disease caused by an enlarged heart.

      e. Increased pulsations in the epigastric area often caused by pulsations of the abdominal aorta after exertion.

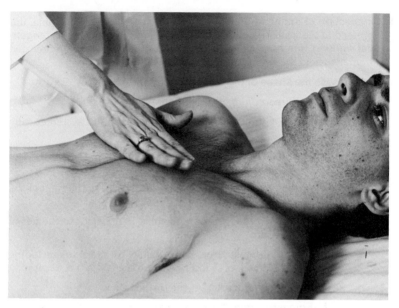

Figure 9–4. Palpation of the precordium using the palmar base of fingers.

Low-frequency vibrations are often easier felt than auscultated.

Thrills. Palpable vibrations (like the purring of a cat) caused by increased blood flow through the heart, distended blood vessels, or diseased valves. Thrills are often associated with grade IV/VI murmurs.

Pulsations. The palpable throbbing of cardiac contractions.

Stenosis. Narrowing of the lumen of the valve owing to calcification or thickening of the leaflets.

Aortic aneurysm. Localized, abnormal dilation of the aorta from congenital weakness of the wall or atherosclerosis.

Pulmonary hypertension is most often caused by mitral stenosis or chronic obstructive lung disease.

Friction fremitus (pericardial friction rub). A grating vibration, synchronous with the heartbeat, that is caused by lack of lubrication as the inflamed pericardial layers rub together. To distinguish friction fremitus from pleural friction rubs, have client hold his or her breath; if the sound continues, it is due to the action of the heart.

IV. Palpation of the precordium.° (For **apical impulse,** see **B.**) **Position** client so that he or she is lying supine with the examiner on the right.

A. **Palpate those areas inspected in III., confirming areas of suspected anomalies.**

   1. **Technique.** Use palmar bases of fingers of right hand to locate vibrations (Fig. 9–4). Move pads of middle and index fingers over precise area. Methodically palpate from base to apex of heart.

   2. **Note** location (in centimeters, from midsternal line), diameter (in centimeters), timing (in relation to the cardiac cycle), ***thrills,*** and ***pulsations.***

   3. **Normal findings**

      a. **Sternoclavicular area** (area around upper sternum). Slight pulsations.

      b. **Aortic area.** No pulsations.

      c. **Pulmonic area.** No pulsations.

      d. **Right ventricular area.** Slight pulsations in thin persons.

      e. **Ventricular area.** Slight pulsations.

      f. **Epigastric area** (under xiphoid process). Slight upward thrust of aorta, usually after strenuous exercise.

   4. **Clinical alterations**

      a. **Sternoclavicular area**

         (1) Pulsations owing to diseases of the thoracic aorta.

         (2) Thrill associated with ***stenosis*** of the carotid artery or heart murmur.

      b. **Aortic area**

         (1) Increased pulsations from ***aortic aneurysm*** or aortic hypertension.

         (2) Thrill associated with stenosis of the abdominal aorta or heart murmur.

      c. **Pulmonic area.** Increased pulsations from pulmonary hypertension° or an aneurysm at the base of the aorta.

      d. **Right ventricular area.** Increased pulsations from a ventricular aneurysm or a right ventricular thrust.

      e. **Epigastric area.** Increased pulsations owing to an abdominal aneurysm or aortic regurgitation.

      f. ***Friction fremitus*** often from pericarditis.

Apical impulse. The most lateral pulsation of the left ventricle noted over the apex of the heart, previously called the point of maximal impulse.

If unable to palpate the apical impulse, have client lean forward causing the heart to fall forward against the chest wall; the exact position of the apical impulse, however, will be altered.

The apical impulse is easier to palpate on forced expiration because less air is in the lungs.

The diameter of the apical impulse depends on the force and volume of ventricular systole.

The amplitude of the apical impulse depends on the thickness of the chest wall and the character of the overlying lung tissue.

Lift. Apical impulse larger than 2 cm.

Heave. Large impulse that actually pushes out against the palpating hand of the examiner.

Increased amounts of air in the emphysematous lung create a cushion between the palpating fingers and the apical thrust.

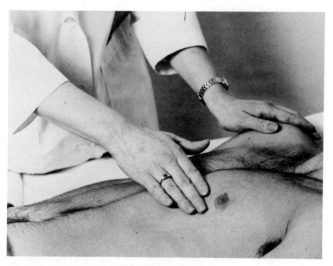

Figure 9–5. Palpation of the apical impulse.

B. **Assess the *apical impulse.***

　　1. **Technique.** Use palmar bases of the fingers of right hand to locate the apical impulse.° Move pads of middle and index fingers over precise area.

　　2. **Instructions to client.** At certain times be prepared to exhale forcibly.°

　　3. **Note** location (in centimeters), diameter,° duration, and amplitude.° Note *lift* or *heaves.*

　　4. **Normal findings.** Apical impulse found in 25 percent of all adults. It is easily located in children and thin adults.

　　　　a. **Location.** Three to 3½ inches (7–9 cm) from midsternal line (Fig. 9–5).

　　　　b. **Diameter.** Less than three-quarters inch (2 cm) (smaller than a nickel).

　　　　c. **Duration.** First third to half of systole.

　　　　d. **Amplitude.** Brisk tap with withdrawal.

　　5. **Clinical alterations**

　　　　a. Apical impulse pushed toward the left often from left ventricular hypertrophy or a right pneumothorax.

　　　　b. Apical impulse pushed toward the right often from right pleural effusion or a left pneumothorax.

　　　　c. Decreased impulse often associated with emphysema.°

　　　　d. Lift or heaves associated with increased volume and pressure in the ventricles.

The cardiac borders are often assessed by the more reliable chest x-ray study; the fingers, however, are more accessible.

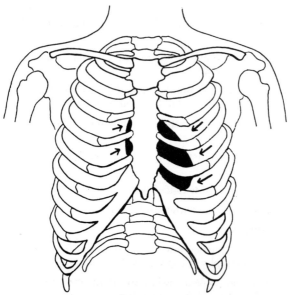

Figure 9–6. Direction of and areas for percussion of the cardiac borders.

Relative cardiac dullness. The dull area of the left side of the heart that retains some resonance owing to the overlying lung tissue.

The position of the trachea must be assessed to determine any deviation from a mediastinal shift.

To accurately interpret findings, the direction of right and/or left shifts must be correlated to each other, as well as any deviation of the trachea.

Mediastinal shift. Movement of the contents of the thoracic mediastinum to the right or left from pulmonary disease.

The traditional auscultatory areas have been extended to correlate more exactly to the origin and transmission of heart sounds.

Left lateral decubitus. Client lying on left side with right knee drawn up.

Mouth breathing increases breath sounds making cardiac auscultation more difficult.

V. Percussion of the cardiac borders.° Determine the location of the cardiac borders.

   A. Position. Client supine with left arm placed behind neck.

   B. Equipment. Skin-marking pencil.

   C. Instructions to client. To women: hold left breast up, away from area being percussed.

   D. Technique. Direct percussion. Using the index finger of the right hand, directly tap the skin. Use very light percussion and begin at the fifth interspace at the left anterior axillary line (Fig. 9–6). Progress medially toward the sternum, moving at small intervals. Repeat procedure in the fourth and then in the third interspace. Mark areas where percussion note changes from lung resonance to *relative cardiac dullness.* Repeat on right side of thorax to assess right cardiac borders.

   E. Note the distance (in centimeters) from the midsternal line of the areas marked in each interspace. Note position of the trachea.°

   F. Normal findings

      1. Left cardiac border. Two to 5 inches (6–12 cm) from midsternal line.

      2. Right cardiac border. Below the right sternal border.

   G. Clinical alterations°

      1. Left border displaced to the left owing to left ventricular hypertrophy, *mediastinal shift* to the left, pregnancy, or cirrhosis.

      2. Left border displaced to the right from a mediastinal shift to the right associated with pulmonary disease.

      3. Right border displaced to the left from pulmonary disease.

      4. Right border displaced to the right from dilatation of the heart or pulmonary disease.

      5. Deviation of the trachea to the side of a mediastinal shift.

VI. Auscultation of the heart.° The **position** of the client varies depending on which area is being auscultated. Supine: all sounds; *left lateral decubitus:* apical sounds, S_3, and S_4; sitting: aortic and pulmonic areas; leaning forward: sounds and murmurs from base. The examiner is on the client's right. Client breathes normally through nose.° Eliminate all extraneous sounds. Necessary **equipment** is a stethoscope (see Chap. 8).

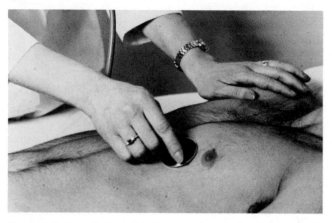

Figure 9–7. Auscultation of the heart at the apical area using the diaphragm of the stethoscope.

Bradycardia. Heart rate of less than 60 beats per minute.

Tachycardia. Heart rate of more than 100 beats per minute.

Heart sound. Previously associated only with the closure of specific valves, heart sounds now include vibrations produced from all the cardiac events and influenced by the viscosity and velocity of the blood, the elasticity of the valves, and the distension of the cardiac chambers.

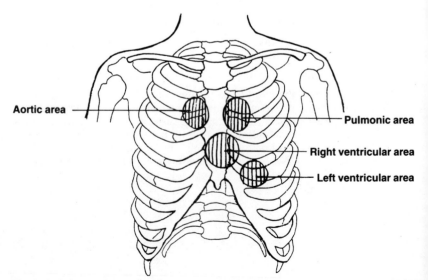

Figure 9–8. Areas of auscultation.

A. **Identify the rate and pattern of the heart beat.**

　1. **Position.** Client supine.

　2. **Technique.** Place diaphragm of stethoscope over apical area and time for 1 full minute (Fig. 9–7).

　3. **Note** rate, rhythm, and variations with respiration.

　4. **Normal findings.** Regular rate is 60 to 100 beats per minute. *Bradycardia* found in highly trained athletes.

　5. **Clinical alterations**

　　a. Bradycardia associated with sick sinus syndrome.

　　b. *Tachycardia* associated with anxiety, thyrotoxicosis, fever, pregnancy, or anemia.

B. **Determine the characteristics of *heart sounds.***

　1. **Technique.** Concentrate on the four areas of auscultation (Fig. 9–8). First auscultate all areas using the diaphragm and then the bell of the stethoscope with client supine, then sitting upright.

　2. **Note** sound, location, pattern, timing, intensity, pitch, splitting, or abnormal sounds.

　3. **Normal findings**

　　a. **Aortic area.** Closure of the aortic valve.

　　b. **Pulmonic area.** Closure of the pulmonic valve.

　　c. **Right ventricular area.** Closure of the tricuspid valve.

　　d. **Left ventricular area.** Closure of the mitral valve.

Note: If anomalies are suspected, assess each sound separately. If none, proceed to I.

S₁. The first heart sound. It is the beginning of ventricular systole and marks the onset of mitral and tricuspid closure (M_1 and T_1).

The identification of S_1 can be aided by placing a finger over the apical impulse because they occur simultaneously.

Closure of the mitral valve precedes the tricuspid but they are so close they are normally heard as one sound.

S_1 is accentuated when the mitral valve remains open at the onset of systole causing it to slam shut.

S_1 is diminished when the heart is weakened or when a fibrosed mitral valve causes limited motion.

S_1 is split when the mitral valve closes before the tricuspid valve.

Ejection click. The audible opening of the pulmonic and/or aortic valves, occurring during systole. Opening of valves is normally silent.

The more common aortic ejection click does not vary with respirations; pulmonic ejection clicks increase with expiration and decrease with inspiration.

S₂. The second heart sound. The vibrations of the blood as it decelerates causes the closure of the aortic and pulmonic valves (A_2 and P_2), signifying the end of systole and the beginning of diastole.

The identification of S_2 can be aided by palpating the carotid impulse while simultaneously auscultating the base of the heart because it is synchronous with the wave of the carotid pulse.

C. Assess the first heart sound (**S_1**).

1. **Technique.** Firmly place the diaphragm of the stethoscope at the apex to identify S_1.° Auscultate all areas systematically progressing toward the base. Repeat using the bell lightly placed on the chest.

2. **Note** sound, location, timing, intensity, pitch, and splitting.

3. **Normal findings**

    a. **Sound.** "Lubb." °

    b. **Location.** Maximum intensity in the mitral and tricuspid areas. Sound is heard in all areas.

    c. **Timing.** Longer than S_2; systole immediately precedes apical impulse.

    d. **Intensity.** Louder at the apex.

    e. **Pitch.** Low.

    f. **Splitting.** Physiologic, heard over the right ventricular area.

4. **Clinical alterations**

    a. Accentuated S_1° often found with hyperkinetic states or mitral stenosis.

    b. Diminished S_1° often found with mitral regurgitation or first-degree heart block.

    c. Split associated with pulmonary hypertension° or right bundle branch block.

D. Identify the presence of an *ejection click.*

1. **Position.** Left lateral decubitus position may help accentuate.

2. **Technique.** Auscultate the apex of the heart using the diaphragm of the stethoscope.

3. **Note** sound (high pitched, clicky), timing (early, mid, or late), and location.

4. **Clinical alterations**

    a. Aortic ejection click° associated with aortic hypertension, aortic valve stenosis, aortic regurgitation, coarctation of the aorta, or hypertension.

    b. Pulmonic ejection click associated with pulmonic valve stenosis or pulmonary hypertension.

E. Assess the second heart sound (S_2).

1. **Technique.** Firmly place the diaphragm of the stethoscope at the base to identify S_2.° Auscultate all areas progressing toward the apex. Repeat using the bell placed lightly on the chest.

2. **Note** sound, location, timing, intensity, pitch, and splitting (in relation to respirations).

Physiologic splitting of S_2 is accentuated on inspiration because the increased venous return to the right side of the heart causes delayed closure of the pulmonic valve. Normal expiratory splitting disappears when the client sits upright.

In mild thickening of valves the valves tense and vibrate; in marked thickening the calcified valve loses its ability to vibrate.

Pathologic splitting heard in the adult (particularly more than 50 years of age) who is erect is an indication of the presence of heart disease.

Wide splitting on inspiration is often caused by delayed electrical activation or atrial septal defect when the ventricle is emptying or contracting.

Fixed splitting does not vary with respiration. Paradoxical splitting widens during expiration and disappears during inspiration.

Opening snap. The audible opening of the mitral and tricuspid valves early in diastole in the presence of pathologic changes within those valves. Opening of valves is normally silent.

Opening snap may be confused with a split S_2 because it appears right after S_2.

S_3 (ventricular gallop). Vibrations caused by rapid diastolic filling of the ventricles, occurring shortly after S_2. S_3 may disappear when client sits up.

3. Normal findings

    a. Sound. "Dupp."

    b. Location. Maximum intensity in aortic and pulmonic areas; heard over all areas.

    c. Timing. Diastole; shorter than S_1.

    d. Intensity. Louder at base. Aortic closure, or A_2, is equal in intensity to pulmonic closure, or P_2.

    e. Pitch. Higher than S_1.

    f. Physiologic split° on inspiration over the pulmonic area in all children and most adults.

4. Clinical alterations

    a. Accentuated S_2 with mild stenosis of aortic or pulmonic valves or pulmonary hypertension.°

    b. Decreased S_2 with marked stenosis of the aortic or pulmonic valve.

    c. Pathologic splitting.°

        (1) Wide split associated with right bundle branch block.°

        (2) Fixed split associated with an atrial septal defect or pulmonary stenosis.°

        (3) Paradoxical split associated with left bundle branch block.

F. Identify the presence of an *opening snap.*

1. Technique. With the diaphragm of the stethoscope, auscultate area medial to the apex and along the left sternal border.

2. Note sound (high pitched and snappy), location (left sternal border), and timing (early diastole).°

3. Normal findings. None.

4. Clinical alterations

    a. Stenosis of the mitral valve and, less commonly, the tricuspid valve.

    b. Abnormally rapid blood flow in conditions such as thyrotoxicosis, mitral regurgitation, and congenital heart defects.

G. Determine the presence of a third heart sound (S_3).

1. Technique. Lightly place bell of the stethoscope over apex. Inch from apex to assess any radiation.

2. Position. Left lateral decubitus.

3. Note sound ("lubb-tup-puh"), location (over apex), timing (early diastole), and intensity (dull, low pitched).

Physiologic S₃. An extra heart sound that is normal and not related to pathology.

S_4 (atrial gallop). Caused by vibrations in the ventricles in response to increased resistance to ventricular filling as the atria contract at the end of diastole. (Eighty percent of the ventricles are passively filled.)

An S_4 may be confused with a split S_1 (must listen attentively for the dull sound of S_4 and the crisper sound of S_1).

Physiologic S₄. An extra heart sound that is normal and not related to pathology.

S_4 is associated with pressure overload of the ventricles and may be accompanied by a palpable extra impulse at the apex.

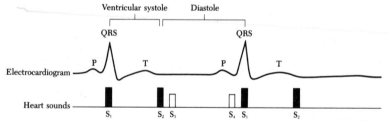

Figure 9–9. Heart sounds in relation to the cardiac cycle and the electrocardiogram. (S_1 = first heart sound; S_2 = second heart sound; S_3 = third heart sound; S_4 = fourth heart sound.)

4. **Normal findings.** None. A *physiologic S_3* may normally be heard in children and young adults, especially after exercise or during periods of stress.

5. **Clinical alterations**

   a. The presence of S_3 is an important sign in the diagnosis of congestive heart failure.

   b. An S_3 in adults is pathologic and usually indicates myocardial failure or mitral regurgitation.

H. **Determine the presence of a fourth heart sound (S_4).**

1. **Technique.** Place bell of stethoscope over medial apex. Inch stethoscope to assess any radiation.

2. **Position.** Left lateral decubitus.

3. **Note** extra beat (very rare), sound,° location (medial to apex), timing (late diastole [presystolic]), and intensity (higher pitched than S_3).

4. **Normal findings.** None. A *physiologic S_4* may be heard in children but is rarer than S_3.

5. **Clinical alterations°**

   a. Frequently heard with cardiovascular hypertension and aortic or pulmonic stenosis.

   b. Summation gallop is sum of S_3 and S_4 found in acute myocardial disease and produces a "lubb-tup-da-da."

I. **Relate normal heart sounds to the presence of abnormal heart sounds.**

1. **Technique.** Identify S_1 and S_2. Relate any other sounds identified previously to S_1 and S_2.

2. **Note** all sounds in relation to each other. A diagram is helpful (Fig. 9–9).

Murmurs. Turbulent vascular sounds that produce vibrations within the heart or the walls of the vessels commonly associated with regurgitation or stenosis.

Standing decreases blood pooled in the cardiopulmonary bed and may eliminate or decrease murmurs.

Table 9–1. Murmur Grades

Grade	Description
I/VI	Soft, barely audible
II/VI	Quiet, but easily heard
III/VI	Quickly audible
IV/VI	Loud, accompanied by a thrill
V/VI	Heard with one side of the stethoscope tilted off the chest
VI/VI	Heard without a stethoscope

Innocent murmurs. Vibrations in normal valves owing to rapid blood flow.

A murmur in children that radiates or occurs in diastole should be carefully assessed.

Pansystolic murmur (holosystolic). Murmur heard throughout systole produced by flow of blood from a high pressure of the ventricle to the low pressure of the atria.

Systolic ejection murmur. Vibrations owing to the ejection of blood from the ventricles into the pulmonary artery or aorta.

Systolic regurgitant murmur. Vibrations owing to the regurgitation of blood from the ventricles into the atria.

Diastolic insufficiency murmur. Vibrations owing to the failure of the aortic or pulmonic valves to close completely.

Diastolic filling murmur. Vibrations owing to the filling of the ventricle through diseased mitral or tricuspid valves.

J. Identify the presence of heart *murmurs.*

  1. Position. Client lying supine.°

  2. Technique. Auscultate all areas first with the bell and then with the diaphragm. If a murmur is present, inch stethoscope to detect any radiation.

  3. Note grade (Table 9–1) or intensity, location, radiation, timing (early, mid, or late systole or diastole), character (crescendo or decrescendo), quality (blowing, harsh, rumbling), pitch (high, medium, or low), variation with respiration, or radiation to the carotids.

  4. Normal findings. None. Young adults or children may have ***innocent murmurs.***°

  5. Clinical alterations

    a. *Pansystolic murmur* associated with mitral or tricuspid regurgitation or a ventricular septal defect.

    b. *Systolic ejection murmurs* associated with aortic or pulmonic stenosis.

    c. *Systolic regurgitant murmur* associated with mitral or tricuspid insufficiency or ventricular septal defect.

    d. *Diastolic insufficiency murmur* associated with aortic or pulmonic insufficiency.

    e. *Diastolic filling murmur* associated with mitral or tricuspid stenosis.

Systolic blood pressure. Measurement of the stroke volume and the pressure exerted against the arterial walls of the aorta.

Diastolic blood pressure. Measurement of blood vessel resistance.

Cuffs that are too small give falsely elevated pressures.

Tucking the stethoscope under the blood pressure cuff may secure the stethoscope, but it falsely elevates the blood pressure.

Blood pressure sounds are low and are best auscultated with the bell of the stethoscope.

Blood pressure should be auscultated down to zero to listen for the the presence of an auscultatory gap.

Korotkoff sounds. Audible vibrations of pressure within an artery. The four phases are as follows:

Phase	Description
1	Beginning of faint sound (systolic blood pressure)
2	Swishing sound
3	Loud, crisp sound
4	Cessation of sound (diastolic blood pressure)

Pulse pressure. Numerical difference between systolic blood pressure and the diastolic blood pressure.

Table 9–2. Causes of Marked Asymmetry (> 10 Torr Difference) in Blood Pressure of the Arms

Errors in measurement
Thoracic outlet syndromes (e.g., cervical rib)
Embolic occlusion of an artery
Dissection of the aorta
External arterial occlusion (e.g., tumor, hematoma)
Atheromatous occlusion
Coarctation of the aorta
Marked difference in arm size (e.g., secondary to unilateral edema or withered arm)
Takayasu's arteritis
After Blalock-Taussig surgical procedure

VII. Examination of the peripheral vascular system.

A. Measure the arterial *systolic blood pressure* and *diastolic blood pressure*.

1. **Equipment.** Stethoscope and sphygmomanometer.

2. **Position.** Client seated comfortably with arm resting on table, raised to heart level; clothing removed from upper arm.

3. **Technique.** place cuff snugly around upper arm, centering air bag over brachial artery. The width of the cuff should be 20 percent of the arm circumference.° The edge of the cuff should be 1 to 2 inches (2–5 cm) above the antecubital space. Do not tuck stethoscope under cuff to secure.° Palpate radial pulse. Inflate cuff 30 to 40 mmHg above point at which palpable artery disappears. Place bell of the stethoscope° over the brachial artery in the antecubital space. Slowly drop pressure to zero,° approximately 3 mm per second. Completely deflate and remove from arm. Listen for **Korotkoff sounds.** Repeat in opposite arm.

4. **Note** systolic blood pressure—level at which sound is first heard—and diastolic blood pressure—level at which last sound is heard. Note *pulse pressure.*

5. **Normal findings.** Blood pressure varies with age; it may be slightly higher in women. Lower limit is 90/60 mmHg and the upper limit is 140/90 mmHg in adults. Pulse pressure is 30/40 mmHg. Systolic pressure in both arms may vary from 5 to 10 mmHg.

6. **Clinical alterations**

   a. Systolic hypertension from an increased stroke volume or rigidity of large arteries associated with atherosclerotic heart disease.

   b. Diastolic hypertension owing to increased peripheral resistance or narrowing of blood vessels.

   c. Decreased pulse pressure from a decreased stroke volume, increased peripheral resistance, or hypovolemia.

   d. Asymmetry in blood pressure of the arms (Table 9–2).

   Note: If client relates any episode of syncope or dizziness or is on an antihypertensive medication, proceed to B. If not, go on to C.

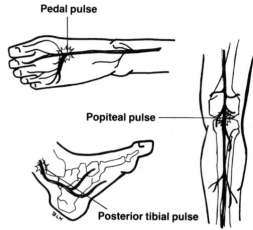

Pedal pulse

Popiteal pulse ──

Posterior tibial pulse

Figure 9–10. Arterial pulses of the lower extremities.

Peripheral arterial pulses are reliable indicators of vascular function.

Pressure applied too firmly over an artery may occlude weak or small vessels, obliterating the pulse.

The carotid arteries are major vessels and, therefore, are accurate indications of arterial pulsations. Carotid arteries should be gently palpated to avoid stimulating the carotid pressoreceptors. Palpating both carotids simultaneously should be avoided because it may cause dizziness, particularly in the geriatric client.

When locating the femoral and popliteal arteries, it is important that the muscles be relaxed to palpate deeply.

The dorsalis pedis or the posterior tibial pulse may be congenitally absent; both, however, rarely are absent.

Grading of Strength

    0 = no pulse

    1 = barely palpable pulsation

    2 = weak pulsation

    3 = strong pulsation

    4 = full and bounding pulsation

B. **Measure postural signs.**

1. **Position.** Client supine, then standing.

2. **Technique.** Apply cuff as in **VII.A.3.** Measure blood pressure as client lies supine. Next, measure blood pressure when client stands.

3. **Note** blood pressure in both positions. Record and compare readings.

4. **Normal findings.** Blood pressure remains the same or may drop a maximum of 10 mmHg systolic and 5 mmHg diastolic.

5. **Clinical alteration.** Postural hypotension associated with the use of antihypertensive medications or prolonged recumbency.

C. **Palpate arterial pulses**° (Fig. 9–10).

1. **Technique.** Place pads of middle fingers over artery to be palpated; vary pressure. Press more firmly with obese or muscular clients.° Simultaneously palpate the corresponding artery on the opposite side of the body. Hold for 15 to 30 seconds. Progress in the following sequence:

    a. **Temperal artery.** Over temporal bone in temple area.

    b. **External carotid.** In the groove between the trachea and the sternocleidomastoid muscle in the middle of the neck region.°

    c. **Brachial.** In the groove between the biceps and the triceps muscles in the inner aspect of the upper arm.

    d. **Radial.** The medial aspect of the arm at the wrist over the radius on the thumb side.

    e. **Ulnar.** The lateral aspect of the arm at the wrist over the ulnar bone on the little finger side.

    f. **Femoral.** In the groin, midway between the anterior superior iliac crest and the symphysis pubis.°

    g. **Popliteal.** Behind the knee, medial to the midline of the popliteal fossa.

    h. **Dorsalis pedis.** On the dorsum of the foot, above the second and third toes, along the extensor tendon of the big toe.°

    i. **Posterior tibial.** In the inner aspect of the ankle, between the medial malleolus and the Achilles tendon.

2. **Note** rate, rhythm, amplitude, quality, strength,° contour, and symmetry.

3. **Normal findings.** Rate between 60–100 in adults. Symmetrical, regular, strong, +3, smooth and rounded.

Tachycardia. Pulse rate of more than 100 beats per minute.

Bradycardia. Pulse rate of less than 60 beats per minute.

Paradoxical pulse. Diminished pulse during inspiration.

Jugular venous pressure. Pressure within the jugular veins. Jugular pulsations reflect atrial contractions; therefore, jugular venous pressure is a good indicator of cardiac arrhythmias.

When client stands or sits erect, gravity causes the column of blood in the jugular veins to fall below the clavicle; when client is supine, the jugular veins are full.

The internal jugular veins give a more accurate pressure reading than the more visible external jugulars.

A change in the jugular venous pressure is especially apparent when compared to a number of previous readings.

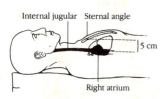

Jugular venous pressure cannot be measured (in supine patient)

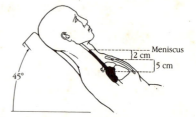

Jugular venous pressure is 7 cm of water

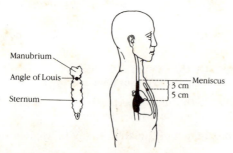

Jugular venous pressure is 8 cm of water

Figure 9–11. Measuring the jugular venous pressure. The sternal angle (angle of Louis) is a bony ridge palpable between the manubrium and the body of the sternum at the level of the second intercostal space. It is always 2 inches (5 cm) vertically above the mid-right atrium. In any position, therefore, one may measure the distance from the sternal angle to the meniscus of the internal jugular vein and add 2 inches (5 cm) to obtain the jugular venous pressure.

4. Clinical alterations

    a. *Tachycardia* in response to exercise, anxiety, smoking, or cold.

    b. *Bradycardia* in a highly trained athlete.

    c. *Paradoxical pulse* often associated with chronic obstructive lung disease.

    d. Weakened pulse from decreased stroke volume associated with congestive heart failure, shock, or aortic stenosis.

    e. Bounding pulse from fever, anemia, hyperthyroidism, or atherosclerosis.

D. Measure *jugular venous pressure* (Fig. 9–11).

1. Equipment. A centimeter ruler, pencil, and an examining table with a top that raises.

2. Position. Client relaxed supine,° with head turned away from side being examined. Head of the bed is elevated 30 to 45 degrees. Provide tangential lighting.

3. Technique. Observe jugular pulsations and assess the quality of pulsations of the internal jugular vein° seen in the soft tissue above the clavicle. If unable to visualize the column of blood in the jugular vein, instruct client to hold breath and bear down (Valsalva maneuver). If still unable to view pulsations, lower bed until pulsations become visible. Lightly place a pencil on the neck on a horizontal plane from the point where the jugular vibrations cease. Place a ruler on the angle of Louis and extend vertically. Measure in centimeters the vertical point where the horizontal pencil crosses the ruler.

4. Note height of blood in the jugular column above the sternal angle, angle (in degrees) of the height of the bed, quality of jugular pulsations, and any change from previous readings.°

5. Normal findings. Jugular venous pressure found 3 cm above the sternal angle with bed at a 45-degree angle; soft and undulating pulsations.

6. Clinical alterations

    a. Increased jugular venous pressure from hypervolemia, especially congestive heart failure.

    b. Decreased jugular venous pressure from hypovolemia related to dehydration.

    c. Loss of jugular pulsations occurring with atrial fibrillation.

    d. Unilateral distension of the jugular veins from local obstruction.

Note: If the jugular venous pressure is elevated, proceed to E. If not, go to F.

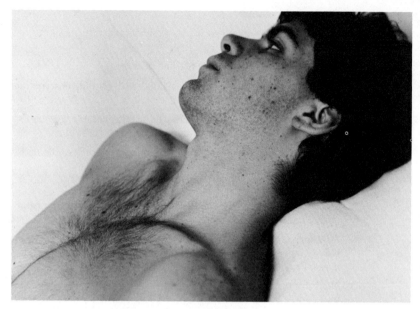

Figure 9–12. Column of blood in the jugular vein.

E. Test the hepatojugular reflux.

1. **Position.** Client lies supine with the head of the examining table elevated so that the jugular pulsations are visible above the clavicle (Fig. 9–12). Examiner is on the client's right.

2. **Instructions to client.** You may feel slight discomfort as I apply pressure over your liver.

3. **Technique.** Place dominant hand over the right upper quadrant and apply firm pressure directed under the ribs, toward the liver.

4. **Note** any increase in the fullness of the veins or rise in the column of blood within the jugular veins.

5. **Normal.** No increase or rise apparent.

6. **Clinical alteration.** Rise in the column of blood owing to hypervolemia within the venous system.

Allen test. Test of the patency of both the ulnar and radial arteries.

The ulnar artery lies deeper than the radial artery and may be more difficult to locate.

The circulation to the hands is protected by the ulnar and radial arteries connected by an arch.

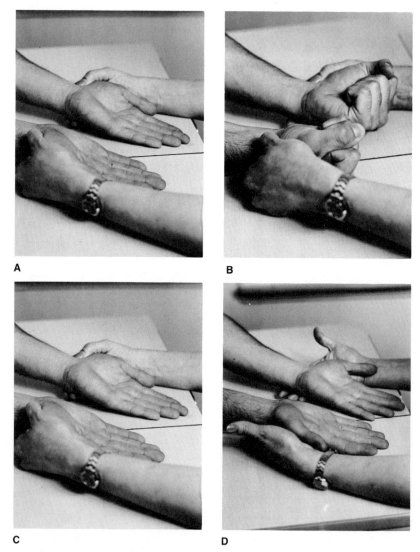

A

B

C

D

Figure 9–13. Allen test. (See **F.3** for explanation.)

F. **Perform the *Allen test*.**

1. **Position.** Client seated comfortably with hands placed on lap.

2. **Instructions to client.** Close hands tightly, making a fist, and hold for 5 seconds as I apply pressure over the arteries in your wrist. Open both hands as directed.

3. **Technique.** Locate ulnar arteries in both wrists.° Simultaneously occlude both arteries by applying firm pressure with thumbs (Fig. 9–13A). Observe palms. Have client close hands tightly, making a fist (Fig. 9–13B). Have client open hands, maintaining pressure on arteries with thumbs (Fig. 9–13C). Release pressure after client opens fists (Fig. 9–13D). Repeat procedure for the radial artery.

4. **Note** rate of the return of normal color to blanched palms with arteries occluded. Note any further change in color once pressure is released.

5. **Normal findings.** Normal color immediately returns as blanched palm is opened.° No increase in color with release of occluded artery.

6. **Clinical alteration.** Pallor of open palm from a vascular insufficiency of the artery not occluded with thumb.

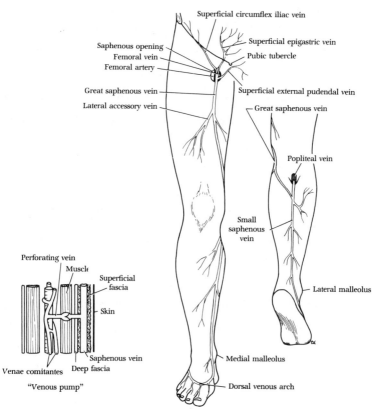

Figure 9–14. Diagrammatic presentation of the venous system in the lower extremities.

The room should be kept warm in order to prevent vasoconstriction from the cold.

A mottled appearance to the extremities may disappear when the client relaxes.

Normal temperature reflects the adequate rate of arterial blood flow through the dermis.

G. **Inspect the legs for venous drainage.**

1. **Position.** Client comfortably seated with arm and leg areas exposed.

2. **Technique.** Systematically inspect the superficial veins (Fig. 9–14).

    a. **Great saphenous.** Extending from the dorsum of the foot up the medial aspect of the leg to the groin.

    b. **Small saphenous.** Extending from the inner aspect of the heel up the side of the leg to the popliteal space where it joins the femoral vein.

3. **Note** nodular, distended veins.

4. **Normal finding.** None. Veins full with legs in dependent position.

5. **Clinical alterations.** Ulcerations, pitting, or thickened skin or cyanosis from venous insufficiency.

H. **Assess circulation: inspect arms and legs for arterial sufficiency.**

1. **Position.** Client seated comfortably with arm and leg area exposed in a warm room.°

2. **Note** color, hair distribution, ulcers, or pulsations.

3. **Normal findings.** Color the same as the rest of the body. No ulcerations or lesions. Decreased amounts of hair in the geriatric client.

4. **Clinical alteration.** Vasoconstriction resulting from anxiety,° a cold room, or arterial insufficiency.

I. **Assess circulation: palpate skin for temperature.**

1. **Technique.** Place back of hand on extremities, beginning at the feet and progressing caudally. Alternate sides.

2. **Note** any difference in temperature of symmetric areas.

3. **Normal.** Temperature is warm on all extremities.

4. **Clinical alteration.** Decreased temperature owing to decreased arterial blood flow.°

Note: If arterial insufficiency is suspected, proceed to J.

Moving the feet when they are elevated helps drain the venous blood from the feet, leaving only the arterial circulation.

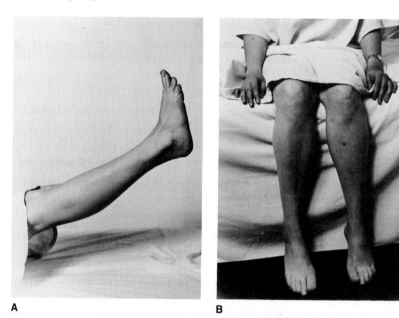

A   **B**

Figure 9–15. Position of the legs during Trendelenburg's test.

Positive Homans' sign. Pain in the calf when the client dorsiflexes the foot.

Lymph nodes. Oval structures, as small as a pin head or as large as a bean, the function of which is filtration and phagocytosis.

Lymph nodes may be palpable in the well person as a consequence of prior inflammation.

Causes of generalized lymphadenopathy:

    Measles

    Systemic lupus erythematosus

    Lymphatic leukemia

    Juvenile rheumatoid arthritis

    Infectious mononucleosis

    Sarcoidosis

J. Perform the Trendelenburg's test.

1. **Position.** Client supine with feet elevated 12 inches (30 cm) above heart.

2. **Instructions to client.** Move feet up and down for 60 seconds when your feet are elevated.° Then, sit up on the table and dangle legs over the edge (Fig. 9–15).

3. **Note** color of feet when elevated and return of color as client sits up and dangles feet.

4. **Normal findings.** Feet pale when elevated with return of normal color when dangling (10 seconds) and filling of veins of feet (15 seconds).

5. **Clinical alterations**

   a. Dependent pallor because of delayed venous filling.

   b. Dependent rubor from arterial insufficiency.

K. Test Homans' sign.

1. **Instruction to client.** Dorsiflex foot with knee slightly bent. Repeat with opposite leg.

2. **Note** pain when foot is dorsiflexed.

3. **Normal finding.** No pain.

4. **Clinical alteration.** *Positive Homans' sign* from deep venous thrombosis.

L. Palpate *lymph nodes.*

1. **Technique.** Use fingerpads of middle two fingers of both hands. Simultaneously palpate and compare contralateral areas. Slowly rotate fingerpads, applying firm pressure.

2. **Note** location, size, tenderness, consistency, and mobility.

3. **Normal findings.** Lymph nodes are not palpable.° Cervical nodes up to 1 cm are often felt in children.

4. **Clinical alterations**

   a. Localized enlargement owing to an inflammation in that area.

   b. Generalized enlargement because of a systemic condition.°

   c. Hard, nontender nodes associated with cancer.

Edema. Excessive accumulation of interstitial fluid.

Pitting. An indentation in the edematous area that persists for a short time after finger pressure is withdrawn.

M. Identify the presence of peripheral *edema*.

    1. Technique. Observe extremities for any swelling. Firmly push thumb over a bone and compress tissue for 5 seconds.

    2. Note *pitting:* location (record in millimeters) and distribution.

    3. Normal finding. No edema.

    4. Clinical alterations

        a. Pitting edema often associated with congestive heart failure.

        b. Peripheral edema associated with lymphatic obstruction, venous disease, or arterial occlusion.

        c. Unilateral edema from a localized cause.

        d. Bilateral edema from a systemic condition.

VIII. Chart

A. Cardiac. Apical pulse 78/min regular; no pulsations or thrills; apical impulse 1.5 cm in diameter, 8 cm from midsternal line, in fifth intercostal space, no heaves or lifts; left cardiac border 3 inches (8 cm) from midsternal line; S_1 and S_2 present; S_2 split on inspiration; no murmurs, gallops, or rubs.

B. Peripheral vascular system. Blood pressure 122/78, right arm, sitting; carotids equal bilaterally; no edema or varicosities; jugular venous pressure 7 cm with bed elevated 45 degrees.

C. Arterial Pulses

	Right	*Left*
Temporal	+3	+3
Carotid	+3	+3
Brachial	+3	+3
Radial	+3	+3
Ulnar	+3	+3
Femnal	+3	+3
Popliteal	+3	+3
Dorsalis pedis	+3	+3
Posterior tibial	+3	+3

Assessment of the Abdomen and Anus

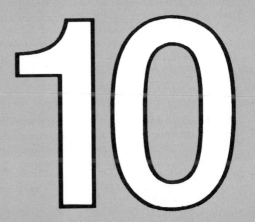

10

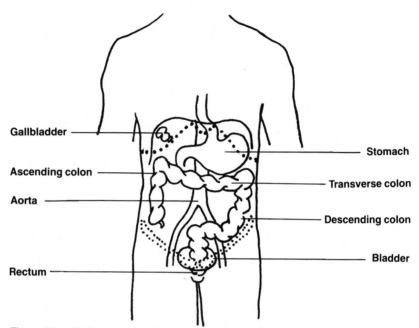

Figure 10–1. Hollow organs of the abdomen. The small intestine is not shown.

Assessment of the cause of pain in the abdomen is difficult. Emphasis must be placed on history and presenting signs and symptoms, particularly location, quality, and pattern of the pain. Acute conditions may require life-saving operations; immediate assessment therefore is vital. Acute conditions include appendicitis, perforated peptic ulcer, dissecting aneurysm, and inflammation or ischemia of an abdominal organ.

Nausea and vomiting. Nausea is the unpleasant sensation before an impending episode of vomiting. ***Vomiting*** is an involuntary act in which violent contractions of the abdominal muscles forcefully move the stomach contents up the esophagus and out of the mouth. Nausea and vomiting are associated with a variety of systemic disorders, most commonly irritative problems of the alimentary canal and peritoneal area. Other causes include nephritis, glaucoma, cerebral lesions, pregnancy (first trimester), and drugs.

Diarrhea. The defecation of loose, watery stools. Defecation is usually frequent with an increase in volume of, and a change in, the characteristics of the stool. Causes include viral gastroenteritis, ulcerative colitis, irritable colon, staphylococcal food poisoning, and dysentery.

I. Examination of the abdomen: General considerations

A. The examiner must possess a thorough understanding of the anatomy and physiology of the abdomen (Fig. 10–1).

B. Assessment of the abdomen differs from other systems. Inspection and auscultation precede percussion and palpation. This sequence delays the more uncomfortable maneuvers until the end of the examination. It also preserves accurate bowel sounds for auscultation. (They may be altered after palpation.)

C. The examiner remains at the client's right (except for special maneuvers).

D. The examination proceeds systematically. Begin in the left upper quadrant and progress clockwise through the remaining quadrants.

E. A warm, relaxed environment is particularly important to promote relaxation of the client.

F. A diagram of the abdomen is an accurate way to chart any anomalies noted.

G. Use a skin-marking pencil for marking on the client.

II. Relevant history questions

A. Pain.° Ask questions related to the following:

   1. Onset, quantity, quality, location, duration, radiation, and history of previous episodes.

   2. Predisposing factors such as stress or activity.

   3. Alteration in dietary pattern such as ingestion of irritating foods.

   4. Associated signs and symptoms such as diarrhea, vomiting, constipation, or indigestion.

   5. Use of therapeutic modalities such as aspirin.

B. *Nausea and vomiting.* Ask questions related to the following:

   1. Onset, quality, duration, color, amount, and consistency of vomitus and history of previous episodes.

   2. Predisposing factors such as foods, smells, or time of day.

   3. Alteration in dietary pattern, foods retained, or anorexia.

   4. Associated signs and symptoms such as pain, diarrhea, indigestion, constipation, or change in weight.

   5. Use of therapeutic modalities such as antacids or antiemetics.

C. *Diarrhea.* Ask questions related to the following:

   1. Onset, duration, type (projectile), number of times a day, color, odor, consistency, and history of previous episodes.

   2. Predisposing factors such as food, fruit juices, or coffee.

   3. Alteration in dietary pattern, weight loss, or anorexia.

Constipation. Infrequent and difficult defecation of hard stools. It is often accompanied by a sense of fullness in the abdomen. The normal pattern for bowel movements varies widely depending on age and life-style. Normal defecation ranges from three times a day to three times a week. Constipation may be due simply to a diet low in crude fiber, inactivity, or laxative abuse; or it may be a clue to an obstruction from a tumor, a neurologic disorder, a local anorectal problem, or an emotional problem.

Indigestion. A substernal, burning, constricting pain usually from an incompetent lower esophageal sphincter that causes reflux of stomach contents to the pharynx. An acid taste is perceived in the mouth, and it often is accompanied by actual regurgitation. Indigestion usually occurs after meals or when the client is lying down. Common causes include peptic ulcer disease, gallbladder disease, and esophageal reflux.

Abdominal distension. An easily recognizable protubant abdomen. There are, however, a variety of causes, which must be explored by palpation and percussion. Common disorders are obesity, feces, pregnancy, neoplasms, tympanites, and ascites.

4. Associated signs and symptoms such as pain, nausea, vomiting, or indigestion.

5. Medications that aggravate such as antibiotics or antacids.

D. *Constipation.* Ask questions related to the following:

1. Onset, duration, color, consistency, and amount of any stools and history of previous episodes.

2. Predisposing factors such as decreased activity, decreased fluid intake, or decreased bulk in diet.

3. Alteration in dietary pattern, anorexia, or weight gain or loss.

4. Associated signs and symptoms such as abdominal pain, nausea, vomiting, indigestion, or abdominal distention.

5. Medications that aggravate such as iron preparations, or antacids.

6. Use of therapeutic modalities such as laxatives or stool softeners.

E. *Indigestion.* Ask questions related to the following:

1. Onset, duration, amount, location, radiation, and history of previous episodes.

2. Predisposing factors such as stress, food irritants, or alcohol.

3. Alteration in dietary pattern such as increased or decreased hunger.

4. Associated signs and symptoms such as belching, flatus, or nausea.

5. Medications that aggravate or relieve such as aspirin or antacids.

F. *Abdominal distension.* Ask questions related to the following:

1. Onset, duration, number of belt holes moved, and history of previous episodes.

2. Predisposing factors such as increased sodium intake, cardiac problems, or alcohol abuse.

3. Alteration in dietary pattern, anorexia, or indigestion.

4. Associated signs and symptoms such as jaundice, pruritus, dyspnea, or swollen hands and feet.

5. Medications that aggravate or relieve such as diuretics, heart medications, or salt pills.

G. **History** of gastrointestinal (GI) problems, past abdominal operations, GI diagnostic procedures, or x-ray studies.

H. **Appetite:** present, recent change, or dental problems.

A warm environment and proper draping promote relaxation of the client and therefore decrease rigidity of the abdominal muscles. If the client is suitably relaxed, the examiner can easily slide his or her hand under the small of the client's back.

Arms folded under the client's head may promote relaxation, but may also tense abdominal muscles.

Deep inspiration may accentuate abdominal pain and cause a "catching" of the client's breath.

Most examiners prefer to divide the abdomen into four quadrants instead of nine areas because the spheres are larger.

Epigastrum. Midline area located directly above the umbilicus.

Aortic pulsations are systolic in timing and are synchronous with the apical impulse.

Diastasis recti. Midline separation of the abdominal rectus muscle.

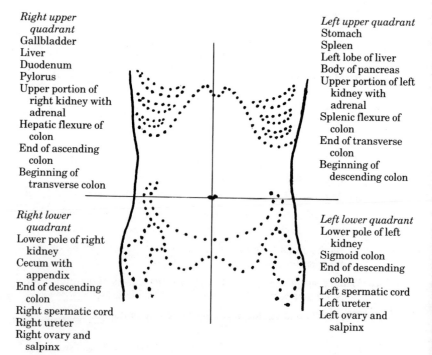

Right upper quadrant
Gallbladder
Liver
Duodenum
Pylorus
Upper portion of right kidney with adrenal
Hepatic flexure of colon
End of ascending colon
Beginning of transverse colon

Left upper quadrant
Stomach
Spleen
Left lobe of liver
Body of pancreas
Upper portion of left kidney with adrenal
Splenic flexure of colon
End of transverse colon
Beginning of descending colon

Right lower quadrant
Lower pole of right kidney
Cecum with appendix
End of descending colon
Right spermatic cord
Right ureter
Right ovary and salpinx

Left lower quadrant
Lower pole of left kidney
Sigmoid colon
End of descending colon
Left spermatic cord
Left ureter
Left ovary and salpinx

Figure 10–2. The four quadrants of the abdomen.

III. **Inspection of the abdomen. Position** client so that he or she is relaxed supine with bladder emptied. Uncover abdomen to symphysis pubis. Drape women's breasts with folded towel. Place small pillow under head. (May also provide a small pillow under knees to further promote relaxation.°) Arms should be either placed along client's side or folded comfortably across client's chest (never under client's head).° Examiner is on right with head slightly above client's abdomen. Provide tangential lighting.

Instruct client to be prepared to inhale and exhale forcibly.°

Each quadrant in turn should be inspected° (Fig. 10–2).

A. **Inspect the *epigastrum* for visible pulsations of the abdominal aorta.**

   1. **Note** location, diameter, duration, direction, and timing (systolic or diastolic) of any pulsations.°

   2. **Normal findings.** Slight, vertical pulsations, systolic in timing, may be seen in thin clients.

   3. **Clinical alterations.** Aneurysm (laterally expansile) or tortuous aorta.

B. **Inspect the abdomen for *diastasis recti*.**

   1. **Instructions to client.** Raise head and hold above pillow for 5 seconds.

   2. **Note** location and length of any separation between the contracted muscles.

   3. **Normal findings.** None.

   4. **Clinical alteration.** Separation of the abdominal rectus muscles from pregnancy, multiparity, congenital weakness, or marked obesity.

C. **Inspect the abdomen for engorged veins and pattern of venous flow.**

   1. **Technique.** Place tips of index fingers in the middle of the visible vein. Push tips apart, "stripping" the vein of blood. Release one finger at a time.

   2. **Note** location of any engorged veins and direction of blood flow (relate to the umbilicus).

   3. **Normal findings.** Faint pattern, visible flowing away from the umbilicus in thin clients.

   4. **Clinical alterations**

      a. Upward filling owing to obstruction of the inferior vena cava or portal vein.

      b. Downward filling from obstruction of the superior vena cava (rare).

Visible peristalsis. Slow undulations seen beneath the contour of the abdomen.

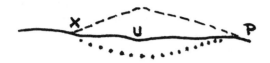

Scaphoid . . .   **Distended — — — —**

Flat _____

Figure 10–3. Contours of the abdomen. (Broken line = distended abdomen; solid line = flat abdomen; dotted line = scaphoid abdomen; X = xiphoid; U = umbilicus; P = symphysis pubis.)

Cullen's sign. Bluish periumbilical discoloration caused by intraabdominal hemorrhage.

Coughing will accentuate the protrusion of an umbilical hernia; tensing of the abdominal muscles may obliterate it.

Sister Mary Joseph's nodule. Umbilical nodule caused by a metastasizing abdominal carcinoma.

D. Inspect the abdomen for *visible peristalsis.*

1. **Note** amplitude and strength of oblique ridges running downward from left to right.

2. **Normal finding.** Slight peristalsis may be visible in thin clients.

3. **Clinical alteration.** Accentuated waves proximal to a partial bowel obstruction.

E. Assess the contour and shape of the abdomen (Fig. 10–3).

1. **Note** lateral slope of the surface of the abdomen from the xiphoid process through the umbilicus to the symphysis pubis.

2. **Normal findings**

   a. **Flat.** Seen in well-developed young clients.

   b. **Round.** Seen in young children and middle-age clients from excess fat or poor muscle tone.

3. **Clinical alterations**

   a. Scaphoid in extremely thin, malnourished, elderly clients.

   b. Distended from ascites.

   c. Round in obese clients or children.

   d. Asymmetry from masses or organomegaly.

F. Assess the umbilicus

1. **Note** position, shape (everted or inverted), color, and character.

2. **Normal finding.** An inverted, oval sphere, vertically placed midway between the xiphoid and the symphysis pubis.

3. **Clinical alterations**

   a. *Cullen's sign.*

   b. Umbilical calculi.

   c. Umbilical hernia.°

   d. *Sister Mary Joseph's nodule.*

   e. Fungal infections.

   f. Tumor displacement.

G. Assess pigmentation.

1. **Note** color of the abdominal skin in relation to the rest of the body, and location, extent, and color of any discoloration.

2. **Normal findings.** Abdominal skin somewhat paler than exposed areas of the body. No discoloration should be present.

Jaundice. A yellowish discoloration from the presence of bile pigments in the skin.

Carotene stains the skin but not the sclera.

Elastic fibers in the reticular layers of the cutis rupture when stretched.

Linea alba. Silvery white line extending from the xiphoid process to the symphysis pubis giving positive evidence of a previous pregnancy.

Hypercorticism causes thinning and increased fragility of the skin.

Old scars are silvery white; new scars are pink or blue. The color of a scar returns to normal in 6 to 8 months.

Keloids. Hypertrophic growth of scar tissue.

The female pattern of hair distribution is triangular with the base at the pubis; the male pattern is diamond with hair growing toward the umbilicus.

The liver fails to conjugate estrogenic substances in advanced liver diseases.

Increased rigidity of abdominal muscles and abdominal distension inhibit abdominal respiratory movement.

Chronic obstructive pulmonary disease accentuates the use of abdominal muscles in the respiratory effort.

3. **Clinical alterations**

   a. Redness.

   b. Ecchymosis.

   c. *Jaundice.*

   d. Carotene° discoloring skin.

H. Inspect abdomen for striae (lines seen after normal skin has been excessively stretched°).

1. **Note** location, color, and length.

2. **Normal findings.** None.

3. **Clinical alterations**

   a. Stretching of the skin from pregnancy (*linea alba*).

   b. Abdominal distension.

   c. Purple lines from Cushing's disease.°

I. Inspect the abdomen for scars.

1. **Note** location, color, length, and character.°

2. **Normal findings.** None.

3. **Clinical alterations**

   a. Traumatic penetration of the abdomen.

   b. Abdominal operations.

   c. *Keloids.*

J. Assess hair pattern (distribution of abdominal and pelvic hair).

1. **Note** texture, amount, and pattern of hair.

2. **Normal findings**°

   a. Women. Scarce abdominal hair; triangular pelvic hair.

   b. Men. Moderate abdominal hair; pelvic, diamond pattern.

3. **Clinical alterations.** Opposite pattern of distribution or change in growth because of hormonal imbalances (adrenocortical or pituitary insufficiency), or liver disease.°

K. Assess respiratory movement (use of abdominal muscles when breathing).

1. **Note** use of abdominal or intercostal muscles during respiration.°

2. **Normal findings.** Men use abdominal muscles; women tend to use intercostal muscles.

3. **Clinical alterations**

   a. Use of intercostals in men owing to abdominal distension.

   b. Use of abdominal muscles in chronic obstructive pulmonary disease.°

Auscultation should always precede palpation because palpation may alter bowel sounds.

Bowel sounds. The audible passage of air and fluid (both are needed to produce a sound) as they move along the lumen of the intestine.

A cold stethoscope or cold hands may stimulate the abdominal muscles to contract.

Optimal area of auscultation. A point in the abdomen to which all bowel sounds are readily transmitted and therefore easily auscultated.

Borborygmi. The loud, long, gurgling sound of hyperactive peristalsis (stomach growling) heard without the use of a stethoscope.

An increased frequency of peristalsis increases the intensity of the sound. Peristalsis of the small bowel is higher in intensity and increases in frequency; the colon is lower, longer, and rambling.

The complete absence of bowel sounds can only be decided after auscultating the abdomen for 5 complete minutes.

A thick abdominal wall (fat or muscle) will decrease the examiner's ability to accurately auscultate the abdomen.

Bruit. A peripheral murmur occurring during systole.

IV. Auscultation of the abdomen.° **Position** client so that he or she is lying supine.

   A. Assess the presence and characteristics of *bowel sounds.*

   1. **Technique.** Lightly place the diaphragm of the stethoscope on the abdomen and systematically auscultate the epigastrum and all four quadrants.° Progress clockwise from the left upper quadrant.

   2. **Alternate technique.** Place the diaphragm of the stethoscope over the *optimal area of auscultation*—a point three-fourths to 1 inch (2–3 cm) below the level of the umbilicus and to the right.

   3. **Note** character, duration, intensity, frequency, and areas auscultated. Relate sounds to time of last meal.

   4. **Normal findings.** High-pitched, irregular gurgles occurring 5 to 34 times a minute.

   5. **Clinical alterations**

      a. Increased peristalsis from ***borborygmi,*** gastroenteritis, diarrhea, early bowel obstruction (proximally).°

      b. Decreased peristalsis from peritonitis, inflammation, paralytic ileus, or late bowel obstruction.

      c. Absence of peristalsis from complete bowel obstruction.°

   B. Identify vascular sounds.

   1. **Technique.** Auscultate all four quadrants,° listening carefully for the following:

      a. Aortic sounds: epigastrum.

      b. Splenic sounds: right and left hypochondria.

   2. **Note** character, timing, location, duration, and intensity of any arterial ***bruits*** or venous hums (rare).

   3. **Clinical alterations.** Aneurysm, hypertension, or renal artery stenosis.

   C. Identify a peritoneal friction rub.

   1. **Technique.** Auscultate all four quadrants using both the bell and the diaphragm of the stethoscope.

   2. **Note** a rubbing, grating sound over the liver or spleen.

   3. **Normal findings.** None.

   4. **Clinical alterations**

      a. Tumor

      b. Abscess of the liver or spleen

Organs lying under the rib cage are usually examined by percussion because they cannot be palpated. Percuss from areas of resonance or tympany to dull because the change in note is easier to assess. Percussion of the abdomen is difficult owing to the many organs and the number of diseases possible.

Tympany usually dominates abdominal percussion because of the presence of gas in the bowel or free floating within the abdomen.

Hollow organs	Solid organs
Stomach	Liver
Intestine	Spleen
Bladder	Pancreas
Colon	Right kidney
Aorta	Left kidney
Gallbladder	Adrenals
	Uterus

Liver span is greater in men than in women.

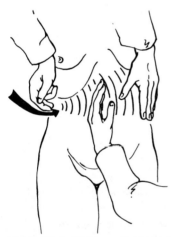

Figure 10–4. Eliciting a fluid wave to demonstrate the presence of intra-abdominal fluid.

If fluid is present, it will create a wave as the fluid transmits the impulse through the abdomen.

V. Percussion of the abdomen.° **Position** client so that he or she is relaxed supine. Necessary **equipment** is a stethoscope.

  A. Compare the distribution of tympany° and dullness of *hollow* and *solid organs.*

    1. Technique. Lightly percuss abdomen in all four quadrants.

    2. Note amount of tympany.

    3. Normal findings. Tympany dominates.

  B. Assess the span of the liver.

    1. Technique. Intermediate percussion in the right upper quadrant and right lower rib cage.

      a. Upper border. Percuss from the third intercostal space down the midclavicular line. Mark area where the percussion note changes from resonance to dull. Repeat this procedure at the midsternal line.

      b. Lower border. Percuss from a level slightly above the umbilicus and up the midclavicular line toward the liver. Mark area where percussion note changes from tympany to dull. Repeat this procedure at the midsternal line.

      c. Note the liver span between the upper and lower borders.°

    2. Alternate technique. Auscultory percussion. Hold stethoscope directly over the liver and lightly scratch with nail toward the liver from all directions. **Note** area over liver where sound intensifies.

    3. Normal findings. Span is 2.5 to 5 inches (6–12 cm) at right midclavicular line; and 1.5 to 3 inches (4–8 cm) at midsternal line.

    4. Clinical alteration. Increased span from fatty infiltration, congestion, portal obstruction, or cancer.

  C. Determine the presence of ascites within the abdominal cavity.

    1. Bulging flanks. Note bulging at either side of the client's abdomen as fluid settles in the dependent flanks.

    2. Fluid wave

      a. Instructions to client. Place ulnar aspect of your arm on your abdomen to prevent any fat from vibrating. May instruct an assistant instead (Fig. 10–4).

      b. Technique. Place palms of both hands on either side of client, midway between lower rib margin and top of the anterior iliac crest. Firmly hit one side, then the other.

      c. Note presence of fluid wave as it travels across the abdomen to the opposite flank.°

Distension of the abdomen is caused by ascites, gas, or obesity. There must be at least 500 ml of fluid to elicit these fluid signs. (The puddle sign may show as little as 120 ml.)

Sound is magnified over a solid organ and diminished over a hollow one.

When turning the client, the air-filled bowel rises to the top and floats; the heavier fluid shifts to the bottom in the direction of gravity pull.

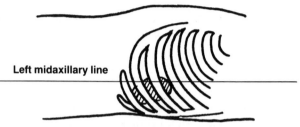

Figure 10–5. Area of splenic dullness.

The spleen is approximately 5 inches (12 cm) long and 3 inches (7 cm) wide. The tympany of the gastric air bubble may interfere with percussion of the spleen.

The splenic percussion note changes to dull when the stomach is displaced by an enlarged spleen.

3. **Shifting dullness**°

    a. Instructions to client. Lie supine until asked to turn to each side.

    b. Technique. Percuss from midsternal line toward one flank, then the other. Mark area where percussion note changes to dull.° Turn client to each side and percuss dependent area, again marking change to dull.°

    c. Note shift in marked fluid line toward the umbilicus, indicating ascites. Measure difference in centimeters. (May elicit a puddle sign with client on all fours. Fluid will puddle in the dependent umbilicus.)

4. **Normal findings.** None.

5. **Clinical alterations**

    a. Ascites from congestive heart failure.

    b. Ascites from the portal obstruction of cirrhosis.

D. Identify area of splenic dullness (Fig. 10–5).

1. **Technique.** Begin at the left anterior axillary line and percuss toward the left posterior axillary line on the 9th, 10th and 11th intercostal spaces.

2. **Note** area where percussion note changes from resonance to dull.

3. **Normal finding.** Area of dullness between the ninth and eleventh intercostal spaces at or posterior to the midaxillary line.

4. **Clinical alterations.** Splenomegaly due to:

    a. Infection.

    b. Hemolytic disease.

    c. Lymphoma.

    d. Cancer of the spleen.

    e. Congestion.

E. Elicit splenic percussion sign.°

1. **Instructions to client.** Be prepared to inhale deeply and hold breath for a few seconds.

2. **Technique.** Percuss lowest palpable interspace in the left lower rib cage at the anterior axillary line.

3. **Note** change in percussion note on full inspiration.

4. **Normal findings.** Percussion note remains tympanic when client inhales.

5. **Clinical alteration.** Dullness on inspiration is indicative of splenomegaly.°

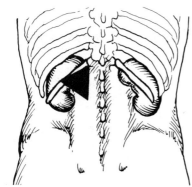

Figure 10–6. Costovertebral angle.

Free air in the stomach will produce tympany.

Normally, the client's bladder will always be emptied prior to the abdominal examination.

Considerations when palpating the abdomen:

Light palpation initially may promote relaxation of the client and prevent involuntary guarding.

Involuntary guarding is a reflex that causes contraction of the abdominal muscles.

Eliminating quick pokes, sharp nails, cold hands, tickling motions, and jarring the bed will decrease the client's anxiety and decrease guarding.

Tender areas should always be examined last.

Rigidity. Tense, boardlike abdomen, which is often indicative of peritonitis.

Cutaneous hyperesthesia. Hypersensitivity of the sensory nerve fibers on the skin.

F. **Elicit costovertebral angle tenderness** (Fig. 10–6).

   1. **Technique.** Place ulnar aspect of fist over area of costovertebral angle. Strike area firmly.

   2. **Note** tenderness over area.

   3. **Normal findings.** No tenderness; will be able to feel the jar.

   4. **Clinical alteration.** Inflammation of kidney.

G. **Identify the gastric air bubble.**

   1. **Technique.** Percuss below the left lower anterior rib cage.

   2. **Note** tympany of gastric air bubble.

   3. **Normal findings.** Tympany in left lower anterior rib cage.°

   4. **Clinical alterations**

      a. Increase in size of the gastric air bubble owing to gastric dilitation.

      b. Displacement of stomach owing to splenic enlargement.

H. **Determine the presence of a full bladder.**°

   1. **Technique.** Percuss area above symphysis pubis.

   2. **Note** circular pattern of dullness.

   3. **Normal findings.** None.

   4. **Clinical alterations**

      a. Distended or full bladder from anuria.

      b. Oliguria.

      c. Urinary retention.

VI. **Palpation of the abdomen.**° **Position** client so that he or she is supine. Examiner is on right, closely monitoring client's expressions for signs of discomfort. If client seems ticklish, begin examination with client's hand under examiner's. **Instruct** client to be prepared to inhale and exhale forcibly using abdominal muscles and to describe any tenderness.

A. **Assess superficial areas.**

   1. **Technique.** Lightly rotate fingerpads in all four quadrants. Abdominal surface should be depressed at least one-third inch (1 cm).

   2. **Note** superficial areas of tenderness, *rigidity,* skin texture, and superficial masses.

   3. **Normal findings.** None.

B. **Test for *cutaneous hyperesthesia.***

   1. **Technique.** Lightly sweep the point of a pin over all quadrants.

   2. **Note** location and extent of pain.

The epigastrum is tender to most clients when palpated. As the abdominal muscles relax and the client gains more confidence in the examiner, deeper palpation can be attempted.

Eighty percent of aneurysms are palpable and are located below the level of the renal arteries. A bruit is often heard over an aneurysm.

The liver descends with the diaphragm on inspiration—it is attached to it by ligaments.

Elevation of the right flank raises the liver toward the anterior abdominal wall.

In bimanual palpation, pressure is exerted by the overlying hand, leaving the lower hand relaxed and sensitive to palpation.

3. **Normal findings.** None.

4. **Clinical alteration.** Increased sensitivity to pain in right lower quadrant from acute appendicitis.

C. **Identify aortic pulsations.**

1. **Technique.** Place palmar surface of the palpating hand in the epigastric area.° Push fingertips inward against the posterior spine. Place middle and index fingertips around precise area of pulsations.

2. **Note** location, timing, character, and direction of pulsations.

3. **Normal findings.** In thin clients, slight pulsations, 1 to 1.5 inches (2.5–4 cm) wide, systolic in timing, may be palpated in the mid-epigastrum.

4. **Clinical alterations**

   a. The lateral pulsations of an aneurysm.°

   b. A tortuous aorta.

D. **Assess the liver as it descends below the rib margin.°**

1. **Technique.** Deep palpation of the right upper quadrant 1½ to 2 inches (4–5 cm) into abdomen. Place thumb side of right hand parallel to the right lower rib margin, fingertips pointing toward xiphoid. Apply firm pressure, pushing in and up under ribs as client inhales deeply. Trace liver edge, if felt, by repeating this procedure both medially and laterally along the contour. (May slide palmar surface of left hand or place a small towel under posterior lower ribs to elevate the flank.)°

2. **Alternate technique.** Bimanual palpation.° For additional pressure, place left hand under right. Maintain position and push deeper as abdomen relaxes after each expiration.

3. **Note**

   a. Client's expression.

   b. Edge of liver as it descends toward examiner's hand as the client inhales.

   c. Tenderness, masses, size, contour, consistency, mobility, and pulsations.

4. **Normal findings.** Not palpable except in thin clients.

Assessment of liver tenderness is assessed by striking the rib cage anteriorly because the liver lies anterior to the kidneys.

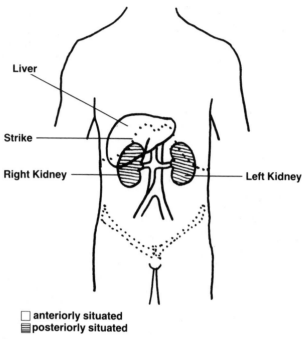

☐ anteriorly situated
▤ posteriorly situated

Figure 10–7. Location of the liver in relation to the kidneys.

The spleen descends with the diaphragm on inspiration because it is attached to it by ligaments.

The spleen is retroperitoneal and must be greatly enlarged to be palpated.

The keys to effective palpation of the spleen are proper instructions to the client with respect to breathing and gentleness by the examiner.

Scale

Slight: 1–4 cm (⅓ to 1½ inches)

Moderate: 4–8 cm (1½ to 3 inches)

Great: 8+ cm (3+ inches)

5. **Clinical alterations**

   a. Enlarged liver from cancer.

   b. Congestion associated with heart failure.

   c. Inflammation from hepatitis.

   d. Hobnail liver of cirrhosis (late).

E. **Elicit tenderness of the liver.°**

  1. **Technique.** Place ulnar aspect of fist over the anterior margin of the right lower rib cage. Strike firmly (Fig. 10–7).

  2. **Note** tenderness.

  3. **Normal findings.** None, only the jarring sensation.

  4. **Clinical alterations.** Tenderness due to:

    a. Inflammation.

    b. Distension of the liver or gallbladder.

F. **Assess the spleen as it descends below left anterior rib margin.°**

  1. **Position.** Client relaxed supine; left lateral decubitus position may facilitate palpation, as spleen falls forward.

  2. **Instructions to the client.** Be prepared to inhale deeply and to describe any tenderness.

  3. **Technique.** Extend left hand across client's abdomen and cup palm around posterior aspect of lower ribs. Elevate anteriorly. Place right hand at an oblique angle, anteriorly, below rib margin. Firmly press both hands together, trying to "capture" the spleen as client inhales. Repeat on either side of initial position.

  4. **Alternate technique.** Examiner on left with client in left lateral decubitus position. Hook fingertips of both hands under left anterior lower rib cage. Press in and up as client inhales.°

  5. **Note**

    a. Client's expression.

    b. Edge of spleen as it descends toward the examiner's fingers as client inhales.°

    c. Tenderness, masses, consistency, mobility, and pulsations.

    d. Size measured in centimeters below rib margin.°

G. **Test for Murphy's sign.**

  1. **Technique.** Hook thumb or fingers under right anterior rib margin as client inhales.

  2. **Note** a painful catch in inspiration as inflamed gallbladder descends over finger.

  3. **Normal findings.** None.

  4. **Clinical alteration.** Inflammation owing to acute cholecystitis.

The following normal structures are often incorrectly assessed as enlarged organs or masses:

1. Twelfth rib
2. Pregnant uterus
3. Full bladder
4. Large amount of feces in the colon
5. Sacral promentory
6. Abdominal aorta

The kidney is not attached to the diaphragm; therefore, it does not move freely with respiration.

The lower pole of the right kidney is lower than the lower pole of the left.

Fluid is more easily displaced than a solid organ or mass.

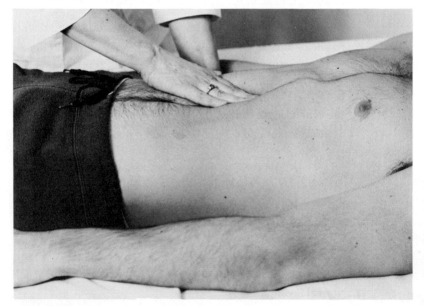

Figure 10–8. Bimanual palpation of the right kidney.

H. **Palpate for an enlarged kidney.**°

1. **Instructions to client.** Be prepared to hold breath on full inspiration. Describe any tenderness.

2. **Technique**

   a. **Right kidney.** Slide left hand under client's right flank (midway between the lower edge of the rib cage and the top of the anterior iliac crest). Elevate flank anteriorly. Place right hand over corresponding anterior surface. Press deeply and try to "capture" kidney below tips of both fingers as client holds breath (Fig. 10-8). Release pressure and allow kidney to slide back into place as client exhales.°

   b. **Left kidney.** Slide left hand across client and under his or her left flank. Elevate anteriorly. Deeply palpate corresponding anterior surface with right hand. (May also "capture" left kidney.)

3. **Note**

   a. Client's expression.

   b. Lower pole of the kidney as it slides back into place as client exhales.

   c. Tenderness, size, contour, mobility, and consistency.

4. **Normal findings.** Kidney not palpable. The lower pole of the right kidney can occasionally be felt in thin clients.°

5. **Clinical alterations**

   a. Enlarged kidney from cysts.

   b. Tumors.

   c. Hydronephrosis.

I. **Assess the presence of a moveable mass.**

1. **Technique.** Hold fingers straight, at a right angle to the forearm. Make a quick thrust toward the mass to be examined.

2. **Note** change in abdominal contour when displacing overlying fluid to reveal a moveable mass against fingers.°

3. **Normal findings.** None.

Appendicitis. Inflammation of the appendix confirmed by the following:

1. Cutaneous hyperesthesia
2. Pain radiating from the umbilicus to McBurney's point (a point located midway between the umbilicus and the right superior anterior iliac crest)
3. Positive psoas sign
4. Muscle rigidity
5. Rebound tenderness
6. Pain in the right lower quadrant (positive Rovsing's sign)

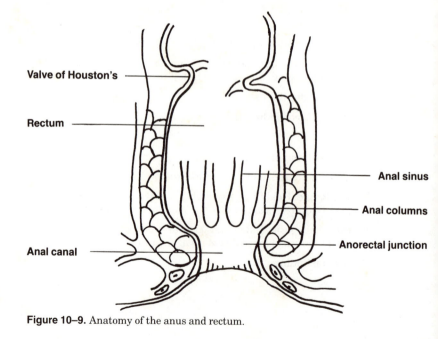

Figure 10–9. Anatomy of the anus and rectum.

J. **Elicit rebound tenderness.**

1. **Technique.** Firmly push palpating hand into the abdomen (not over an area of direct tenderness). Quickly release.

2. **Note** tenderness as the abdomen springs back.

3. **Normal findings.** None.

4. **Clinical alteration.** Tenderness owing to peritoneal irritation from *appendicitis.*

K. **Test for psoas sign.**

1. **Instructions to client.** Flex legs at hips.

2. **Technique.** Alternately place hand above each knee and press firmly.

3. **Note** pain in the left lower quadrant.

4. **Clinical alteration.** Pain from irritation of the lateral psoas muscle owing to an inflamed appendix.

VII. **Examination of the anus: General considerations**

A. The examiner should be thoroughly familiar with the anatomy and physiology of the anus (Fig. 10–9).

B. The rectal examination is never done routinely on children. It should be done once a year in men more than 40 years of age. It is always a part of the routine pelvic examination in women.

C. Gloves should always be worn when examining the rectum.

D. Efforts should be made to relax the client because the rectal examination is uncomfortable and considered invasive and embarrassing.

E. The client should defecate before the examination to clear the anal canal of feces.

The rectal examination completes the examination of the abdomen; it should be performed last.

The left lateral position is the best position to perform the rectal examination on elderly, debilitated, or unconscious clients. In women the rectal examination is best performed in the lithotomy position because it usually follows a pelvic examination.

Classification of hemorrhoids:

Degree	Description
First	Merely bleed
Second	Prolapse when straining but recede spontaneously
Third	Permanently prolapsed

External hemorrhoids are located below the pectinate line and are red, ragged tabs; internal hemorrhoids are located above the pectinate line and are red masses covered with mucosa, which may descend as the client strains.

VIII. Inspection and palpation of the anus and anal canal.° **Position** male client so that he is standing on the floor with his upper trunk lying across the examining table with hips slightly flexed. Women are in lithotomy position. Client is lying on examining table with buttocks at the bottom edge of the table with feet in stirrups and knees flexed and abducted.°

Instruct client to bear down as if he or she is having a bowel movement when asked to do so and to try to relax and describe any tenderness.

A. Inspect the anus and perianal area.

   1. Technique. Place each hand on buttocks and spread to expose anus.

   2. Note color, texture, hair, bulges, and prolapse when the client strains. If hemorrhoids are present, note classification.°

   3. Normal findings. Skin is more pigmented and coarser, sparse amounts of hair. Anus puckered and reddish brown in adults, redder in children.

   4. Clinical alterations

      a. Tuft of hair or dimpling below coccyx commonly associated with a pilonidal sinus.

      b. A perianal rash associated with pruritus ani.

      c. Bulging or protrusion of red mucosa from rectal prolapse or hemorrhoids.°

      d. Fluid-filled vesicles commonly associated with herpesvirus II.

When the examiner's finger is placed on the anus, the sphincter will tighten and then slowly relax.

Insertion of the finger into the anus is not painful if done very slowly and gently. The examiner's nails should be short and care should be taken not to scratch the delicate anal mucosa.

Rectal masses are often malignant.

The anal sphincter may be closed tightly in the client who is very apprehensive. Reassure the client and have him or her take deep breaths to relax.

B. **Palpate the anus and anal canal.**

1. **Instructions to client.** Bear down as examiner's finger is inserted. You may feel pressure as you would if you were having a bowel movement. Tighten sphincter when asked to do so. Describe any tenderness.

2. **Equipment.** Glove or finger cot; lubricating jelly.

3. **Technique.** Using index finger (little finger in children), generously lubricate finger cot or gloved finger. Place finger firmly over anus.° As sphincter relaxes, slowly insert finger through the anus, in the direction of the client's umbilicus.° Evenly rotate finger 360 degrees around rectal walls. Gently withdraw finger and test any stool for occult blood.

4. **Note** tenderness, masses, consistency of rectal wall, lumen of the anal canal, and muscle tone as sphincter closes around finger.

5. **Clinical alterations**

   a. Hard nodules and narrowing of the canal often associated with anal carcinoma.°

   b. Hard mass occluding canal owing to a fecal impaction.

   c. Relaxed sphincter often associated with tabes dorsalis or a spinal cord lesion.

   d. Hypertonia often from tension° or a local irritation such as a fissure.

IX. Chart

A. **Abdomen.** Abdomen flat, symmetric, with inverted umbilicus, centrally located; no diastasis recti, scars, striae, engorged veins, lesions, visible peristalsis, or pulsations; hair pattern triangular; uses abdominal muscles when breathing.

   Bowel sounds normal, 20 to 22 per minute; no bruits or venous hum; no peritoneal friction rub.

   Tympany present in all four quadrants; no fluid wave, bulging flanks, or shifting dullness; liver span 4 inches (10 cm) at right midclavicular line and 1 inch (3 cm) at midsternal line; splenic percussion note tympanic; no costovertebral angle tenderness.

   No tenderness or masses; good muscle tone; liver, spleen, and kidneys not palpable.

B. **Perianal area.** No lesions, rash, inflammation, bulges, or external hemorrhoids.

C. **Anus.** Good sphincter tone; no tenderness or masses; no hemorrhoids or rectal prolapse; rectal mucosa smooth; negative for occult blood.

Assessment of the Male Genitalia and Prostate

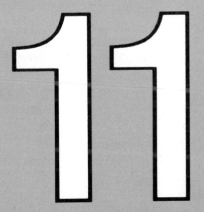

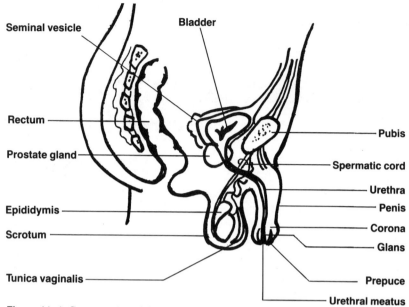

Figure 11–1. Cross section of the male genitalia.

Pain should be identified as low back, abdominal, inguinal, penile, scrotal, testicular, or rectal. Acute conditions requiring immediate care are pyelonephritis, spermatic cord torsion, strangulated inguinal hernia, urinary retention, and gonorrhea. Increased physical activity or straining prior to or increasing scrotal or inguinal pain suggest inguinal hernia.

Discharge is generally copious yellow with gonorrhea; slight watery mucus with nonspecific urethritis; bloody, possibly with hematuria, with urinary tract calculi or trauma.

Onset of symptoms should be correlated to incubation periods of venereal diseases and recent history of trauma, illness, and sexual activity.

Genital lesions

  1. Syphilitic chancre. Painless, round, silvery, or darkened ulcerated lesion usually on coronal sulcus and less frequently on penile shaft or scrotum. Chancre may exude a serous discharge containing *Treponema pallidum*.

  2. Condyloma acuminatum (venereal warts). Villous, warty pointed growths usually noted at corona, which are either single or in groups.

  3. Genital herpes (herpes progenitalis). Group of vesicles or ulcerations on erythematous base occurring frequently on glans or prepuce.

Onset of lesions should be correlated to sexual activity and incubation period of venereal diseases. Vesicular or papular lesions associated with pruritus on penis, scrotum, or in pubic hair may represent scabies infection or phthirus infestation.

I. General considerations

A. A thorough knowledge of the anatomy, physiology, and pathology of the male urinary and reproductive systems is essential (Fig. 11–1).

B. The sequence of evaluation should be obtaining a thorough, detailed history; inspecting and palpating the genitals; transilluminating the scrotum; auscultating a scrotal mass when necessary; and evaluating the prostate gland.

C. The examination varies with patient, chief complaint, and setting.

D. The patient should initially be examined standing on the floor facing a seated, gloved examiner.

E. Environment should be warm and private, ability to darken examination room is helpful.

F. The patient should be verbally instructed throughout the examination regarding maneuvers about to be performed.

G. Adolescent males are sensitive about their changing sexuality. Parents should not be present during the history or physical examination.

H. Health teaching is important to integrate throughout the examination because of the prevalence of venereal disease.

II. Relevant history questions

A. **Pain.**° Ask questions related to the following:

    1. Location, onset, quantity, duration, course, quality, radiation, and history of previous episodes.

    2. Predisposing factors such as increased activity, trauma, or previous symptoms.

B. **Penile discharge.**° Ask questions related to the following:

    1. Onset,° quantity, color, viscosity, and pruritus.

    2. Predisposing factors such as past and present sexual activity, trauma, history of back pain, or fever.

C. **Genital lesions.**° Ask questions related to the following:

    1. Onset, location, tenderness, pruritus, and lesion discharge.

    2. Predisposing factors such as trauma, past and recent sexual activity, history of genital lesions, general medical history, or circumcision.

    3. Associated signs and symptoms such as discharge, fever, dysuria, regional adenopathy (tender and nontender), or oral or finger lesions.°

Sexual dysfunction may result from temporal or spinal cord lesions, diabetes mellitus, tabes dorsalis, previous rectosigmoid operations, vascular disease, genital trauma, psychological disturbance, and medications including antihypertensives, phenothiazines, and methadone. Chronic alcoholism or liver disease contributes to diminished libido, testicular atrophy, and impotence. Disease entities or drug side effects are frequently missed because examiners neglect to question patients concerning sexual functioning.

Scrotal enlargement. Painful unexplained swelling in scrotum that may indicate epididymitis, scrotal hernia, or testicular torsion.

Testicular enlargement. Insidious, persistent testicular enlargement that suggests testicular cancer.

History of recent trauma should suggest hematocele or hydrocele.

Urinary dysfunction:

1. Polyuria (frequent urination) suggests diabetes mellitus, excessive xanthine intake, polydipsia, or infection.
2. Dysuria (difficult urination) suggests mechanical obstruction from urethral stricture, urinary tract calculi, or prostatic enlargement.
3. Painful urination suggests infection in prostate, bladder, or urethra.
4. Hematuria suggests urinary tract calculi, trauma, or malignancy.
5. Dark urine suggests dehydration, trauma, liver disease, hyperbilirubinemia, or glomerulonephritis.

D. **Sexual activity and function.** Ask questions related to the following:

1. History of venereal disease.

2. Past and recent sexual activity.

3. Sexual dysfunction.°

   a. Onset, absence, or presence of erections and ejaculations, libido, orgasm, infertility, and trauma.

   b. General medical history.

   c. Medications.

   d. Stress and emotional conflicts.

E. *Scrotal* **and** *testicular enlargement.* Ask questions related to the following:

1. Location, onset, consistency, and pain.

2. Predisposing factors such as physical activity, disease, or trauma.°

F. **Urinary dysfunction.**° Ask questions related to the following:

1. Onset, urinary frequency, hesitancy, urgency, and urine color.

2. Predisposing factors such as trauma, diabetes mellitus, prostatitis, diet, dehydration, medication, liver or kidney disease, or physical activity.

3. Associated signs and symptoms such as glycosuria, proteinuria, specific gravity increase or decrease, hyperbilirubinemia, rectal or prostatic pain or pressure, low back pain, dependent edema, hematuria, or pyuria.

4. General medical history and past genitourinary surgical history.

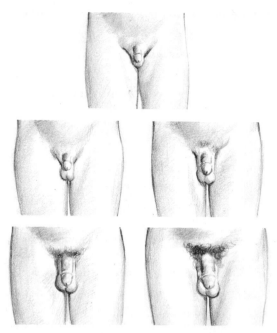

Figure 11–2. Pubic hair and penis development in males.

Phthirus pubis. Crab louse that infests genital region.

Circumcision. Process of surgical removal of prepuce. Carcinoma of penis is limited almost exclusively to men not circumsized in childhood.

Priapism. Prolonged, persistent penile erection without sexual desire.

III. Inspection of the male genitalia. Position client so that he is standing on the floor facing the seated examiner. A warm, private environment with good lighting is essential.

A. Inspect the pubic hair.

1. **Note** presence and distribution and Tanner stage of pubic hair development (Fig. 11–2).

2. **Normal findings.** Diamond-shaped pattern in the adult male. Varies with sexual maturity.

3. **Clinical alterations**

   a. Absent or scant distribution may indicate pituitary or adrenocortical dysfunction or chronic alcoholism with liver disease.

   b. Scattered 1- to 2-mm ova attached to hair shafts with **Phthirus pubis.**

B. Inspect inguinal area.

1. **Note** presence of bulges or surgical scars.

2. **Normal findings.** None.

3. **Clinical alterations**

   a. Inguinal bulging may represent a femoral hernia or inguinal adenopathy.

   b. Surgical scar suggestive of hernia repair.

C. Assess penis.

1. **Note** size, position, pigmentation, **circumcision,** and Tanner staging of genital development (see Fig. 11–2).

2. **Normal findings.** Although wide variation occurs in the normal size of the penis, a marked discrepancy between penile size and patient age warrants further evaluation.

3. **Clinical alterations**

   a. Disproportionately small penis from eunuchism or hypoplasia.

   b. Disproportionately large penis from Leydig cell tumor or **priapism.**

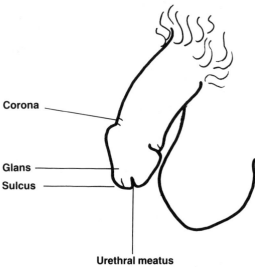

Figure 11–3. Inspection of the corona and sulcus.

Paraphimosis. Inability to reduce retracted foreskin over glans; constriction may result in surgical emergency.

Chancre. Superficial ulcer with serous drainage which is the primary lesion of syphilis. It is commonly found on the corona.

Herpes progenitalis. Small group of vesicles surrounded by erythema. It commonly occurs on the prepuce.

Treponema pallidum (the spirochete of syphilis) may penetrate unbroken skin; examination gloves must always be worn.

Consider Reiter's syndrome in men between the ages of 20 and 24 who have the classic triad of symptoms: urethritis, conjunctivitis, and arthritis.

Both gonorrhea and nonspecific urethritis may be present without discharge or painful urination.

Urethral strictures are usually congenital malformations.

D. Inspect sulcus and corona (Fig. 11–3).

   1. Instructions to client. Retract foreskin (prepuce) from glans.

   2. Note scattered erythematous papules, silvery papules, ulcerations, vesicles, villous projections, and warty growths.

   3. Normal findings. None.

   4. Clinical alterations

      a. *Paraphimosis.*

      b. *Chancre.*

      c. *Herpes progenitalis.*

E. Inspect urethral meatus.

   1. Technique. With gloved hand,° gently compress glans between thumb and second digit to open urethral meatus.

   2. Note discharge quantity and color; obtain sample for laboratory evaluation.

   3. Normal findings. Meatus pink without discharge.

   4. Clinical alterations°

      a. Copious discharge in gonorrhea.°

      b. Scant, clear discharge in nonspecific urethritis.

      c. Tender, erythematous edges of urethral meatus associated with urethritis.

      d. Stricture.°

Absence of the testicle from the scrotum may be congenital (maldescension or cryptorchidism) or from surgical removal.

Exposure to cold shrinks scrotal sac; exposure to warm relaxes and enlarges sac.

Frank edema is caused by hydrocele, hematocele, or other general medical conditions associated with edema.

Sebaceous cysts are the most common scrotal lesions, appearing as scattered, firm, nontender whitish lesions.

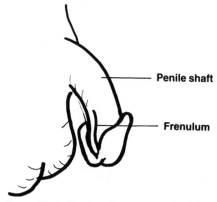

Figure 11–4. The frenulum and penile shaft.

F. Assess scrotum.

   1. Instructions to the client. Please lift scrotum so I can inspect posterior surface.

   2. Note size, prominent bulges, lesions, edema, and rashes.

   3. Normal findings. Soft pouch hanging from base of penis, left side normally lower than right; tissue divided along midline ventrally, each side containing testicle, epididymis, and spermatic cord.

   4. Clinical alterations

   a. Absence of one or both testicles.°

   b. Constricted scrotum.°

   c. Bulging mass associated with scrotal hernia, varicocele, or tumor.

   d. Scrotal edema.°

   e. Sebaceous cysts.°

IV. Palpation of the male genitalia. Position client so that he is standing facing the seated examiner. Provide good lighting and ensure privacy. Examining hand is gloved. **Instruct** client that you are going to gently examine the genitals; it will not be painful.

A. Palpate penis.

   1. Technique. Grasp penile shaft between thumb and index and middle fingers, palpating from scrotum to meatus.

   2. Note nodules, tenderness, plaques, indurations, and consistency of discharge.

   3. Normal findings. Three columns of tissue with two evident dorsally and one ventrally. The frenulum is a fold of prepuce evident ventrally from meatus to neck (Fig. 11–4).

   4. Clinical alteration. Lesions suggestive of venereal disease.

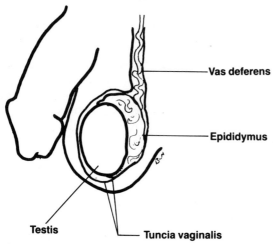

Figure 11–5. The scrotum.

Scrotum. Skin-covered pouch suspended from the perineal region, containing the testes, epididymus, and spermatic cord.

Testes. Small oval glands in the scrotal sac that produce sperm and secrete the hormone testosterone.

Testicular tumor accounts for 12 percent of all deaths from cancer in men between the ages of 15 and 34. It may present as either a firm, stonelike lesion attached to testicular wall or the slow enlargement of a testicle. Testicular cancer is frequently *painless*. Self-examination of the testicles should be taught to all adolescent and adult men during the examination.

Varicocele. A plexus of veins forming a soft, irregular mass in the scrotum generally superior to the testicle and frequently (85 percent of the time) on the left side. It is often described as feeling like a "bag of worms," is nontender, and occurs in 10 to 15 percent of men. Twenty to 40 percent of infertile men have varicoceles, suggesting a relationship. A varicocele is reduceable when patient is standing.

Epididymis. Tightly coiled tube (approximately 20 feet in length) that serves as a duct through which sperm pass.

Seven percent of men have anterior location or anteversion of the epididymis.

Acute epididymitis usually is due to infection or trauma. The testicle may be tender and swollen. Associated symptoms include fever and leukocytosis.

B. **Assess external *scrotum*** (Fig. 11–5).

   1. **Technique.** Spread the scrotal wall tissue between fingers.

   2. **Note** swelling, edema, cysts, and lesions.

   3. **Normal findings.** None. Scrotum may be pendulous in the elderly client.

   4. **Clinical alterations.** Varicocele or hydrocele (especially in children less than 2 years of age).

C. **Examine scrotal contents.** The examination should be performed in the following order:

   1. *Testes*

      a. **Technique.** Gently palpate each testicle between thumb and index and middle fingers. Next, palpate tissue superior to the testicles.

      b. **Note** presence or absence of testicles, size, tenderness, and presence of lesions. Note presence of mass extending toward the inguinal canal.

      c. **Normal findings.** Both testicles descended, testes firm ovoid mass approximately 1 to 1½ inches (3–4 cm) extending vertically suspended by spermatic cord.

      d. **Clinical alterations**

         (1) Firm mass attached to testicular wall.°

         (2) Edematous and tender or nontender testicle.

         (3) Absence of testicle from a congenitally undescended testicle or the surgical removal of one.

         (4) Mass superior to the testicles from a ***varicocele*** or hernia.

   2. *Epididymis*

      a. **Technique.** Gently palpate the upper testicular pole to find soft mass extending posteriorly to lower testicular pole. Palpate in this order: head, body, and tail.

      b. **Note** location,° size, and tenderness.

      c. **Normal findings.** Nontender firm mass.

      d. **Clinical alterations**

         (1) Anterior location of epididymis.

         (2) Enlarged, tender epididymis with epididymitis.°

         (3) Palpable mass with spermatocele or tumor.

Spermatic cord. Contains the vas deferens, nerves, blood vessels, lymphatics, and muscle.

Testicular torsion. The twisting of the spermatic cord. Testicular torsion is a medical emergency requiring immediate consultation. Occlusion of the arterial, venous, and lymphatic flows may result in edema or irreparable tissue damage. The twists may not be palpable, and the hip on the affected side is often held in flexion. Gentle elevation of the scrotum does not alleviate pain as in epydidymo-orchitis (Prehn's sign).

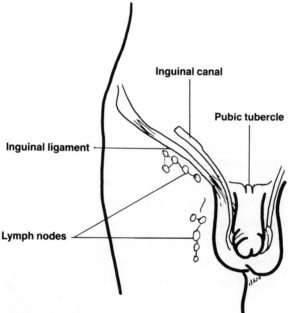

Figure 11–6. The inguinal lymph nodes.

3. *Spermatic cord*

   a. **Technique.** Gently palpate the spermatic cord from the epididymis vertically to the superficial inguinal ring.

   b. **Note** nodularity, tenderness, and masses, comparing right side to left.

   c. **Normal findings.** Vas deferens is a whiplike cord; other structures less definable.

   d. **Clinical alterations**

      (1) Vas deferens or spermatic cord swelling or nodularity suggests syphilis or tuberculosis.

      (2) Soft, irregular mass of vessels between testicle and superficial inguinal ring usually a varicocele.

      (3) Palpable twists in spermatic cord associated with pain or swelling may represent *testicular torsion.*

D. **Examine the inguinal lymph nodes** (Fig. 11–6).

   1. **Technique.** Palpate vertical and horizontal groups of nodes.

   2. **Instruction to client.** Bear down as if moving bowels when told to do so.

   3. **Note** location, size, tenderness, and presence or absence of corresponding nodes on opposite side. Observe change in nodes when client bears down.

   4. **Normal findings.** Horizontal group drains scrotum, penis, skin of lower abdomen, and lower anal canal. Vertical group drains leg. Testicles drain to para-aortic nodes. No enlargement.

   5. **Clinical alterations**

      a. Chronic painless adenopathy may be present in healthy patient and is diagnostically insignificant.

      b. Tender inguinal adenopathy bilaterally in gonorrhea.

      c. Nontender inguinal adenopathy unilateral or bilateral in syphilis.

      d. Usually unilateral tender adenopathy in chancroid.

The inguinal ligament extends from the anterior superior iliac spine to the pubic tubercle. The inguinal canal extends parallel and superior to the inguinal ligament. The lateral opening of the canal joins the abdominal cavity and is located at the inguinal ligaments, midpoint. Approximately 1⅓ inches (3.5 cm) medial and inferior lies the external inguinal ring located in the subcutaneous tissue where the spermatic cord leaves the abdominal muscles.

An indirect inguinal hernia is a mass entering the inguinal canal from the abdominal cavity. It may enter slightly or protrude into the scrotum. It is the most common hernia in both men and women of all ages.

Inguinal canal. Channels piercing the abdominal muscles. In the male, the spermatic cords extend through the canals to the scrotum. The canals are larger in men than in women, accounting for their increased incidence of inguinal hernias.

Femoral hernia. Located approximately 1 inch (3 cm) medial to the femoral artery at the midpoint of the inguinal ligament, a small hernia may bulge anteriorly when patient strains. This bulge distinguishes it from inguinal lymph nodes. Femoral hernias are infrequent, never in the scrotum, and are associated with an empty inguinal canal.

Reduceable scrotal mass. A mass in the scrotum that diminishes or reduces. It may indicate varicocele or hernia. A hernia that is not reduceable is incarcerated.

A hernia is strangulated when circulation is impaired leading to edema, systemic symptoms, and pain.

E. Detect the presence of hernias.° Instruct client to bear down when told to do so.

1. **Assess for scrotal hernia.**

    a. Technique. Patient standing on floor facing seated examiner. Gently grasp the superior aspect of scrotum between thumb and second and third digits.

    b. Note any mass extending into superficial inguinal ring.

    c. Normal findings. No palpable mass.

    d. Clinical alteration. A mass usually represents an indirect inguinal hernia in the scrotum° or varicocele.

2. **Assess *inguinal canal* and femoral ring.**

    a. Instructions to client. Bear down when asked to do so. A child should be told to blow up a balloon.

    b. Technique. Place the tip of the second right finger at the dependent aspect of the scrotum and invaginate the loose tissue proceeding superiorly into the right superficial inguinal ring. Attempt to follow the inguinal canal with the examining finger laterally in an oblique course toward the right anterior superior iliac spine. When resistance is felt, instruct the patient to bear down. Palpate femoral canal area for masses or tenderness. Again, instruct patient to bear down and assess area for bulging.

    c. Note the presence of a herniating mass or bulge felt against tip of examining finger. The procedure is performed identically on the patient's left side using the examiner's left second finger.

    d. Normal findings. No mass is identified. Hernias are fairly common in children.

    e. Clinical alterations

        (1) Small ***femoral hernia.***

        (2) Herniating mass in canal represents a direct or indirect inguinal hernia.

        (3) Mass extending from superficial inguinal canal into scrotum may be ***reduceable.*** To determine, with the patient in a supine position, the examiner should gently attempt to push scrotal mass superiorly toward superficial inguinal ring and abdominal cavity.°

        Note: If any abnormal scrotal masses are found, proceed to F. and G. If not, proceed to V.

Transilluminate. To introduce a light source behind soft tissue in the body to reveal the opacity or translucency of tissue contents.

A herniated loop of bowel into scrotum may transmit peristaltic sounds. Positive findings confirm the presence of herniated bowel. A negative finding, however, does not exclude herniated bowel.

Examination of the rectum and prostate should be performed at least annually in men 40 years of age or older.

F. *Transilluminate* **the scrotum.**

1. **Position.** Patient standing on floor facing seated examiner. Room should be darkened, or genitals shaded significantly.

2. **Equipment.** Penlight.

3. **Technique.** Place light source (penlight or flashlight) directly against posterior wall of scrotum and stretch scrotal mass. Masses that transmit light are translucent and appear as red glow. Masses that are opaque block the light source.

4. **Note** the size, configuration, opacity, and translucency of the scrotal mass.

5. **Clinical alterations**

   a. Translucent scrotal masses suggest hydrocele, spermatocele, or edema.

   b. Opaque scrotal masses suggest testicles, hernias, varicoceles, or solid tumors.

G. Identify loop of bowel herniating into scrotum by auscultation.

1. **Position.** Patient standing on floor facing seated examiner.

2. **Equipment.** Stethoscope.

3. **Technique.** Gently place diaphragm of stethoscope against suspected scrotal mass.

4. **Note** evidence of peristaltic sounds.

5. **Clinical alterations.** Peristalsis owing to a herniated bowel.°

V. Examination of the prostate.°

A. Position. The patient may be examined standing leaning over examining table at waist, or in left lateral decubitis position with hip flexed approximately 90 degrees. Position may be determined by circumstances and personal preferences.

B. Equipment. Examination gloves, lubricating jelly, and materials for occult blood testing.

C. Instructions to client. I am going to examine your prostate gland. This examination is performed through the rectum. It may be uncomfortable.

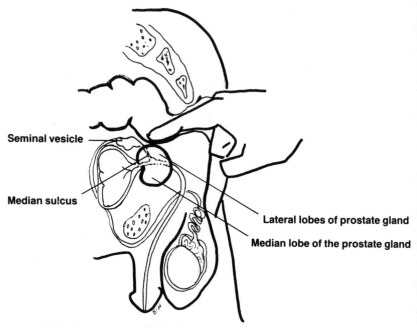

Figure 11–7. Examination of the prostate gland.

A history of difficulty initiating a urinary stream and a sensation of rectal pressure suggests prostatic enlargement.

In men more than 50 years of age, a benign enlargement of the prostate is common. The median sulcus frequently is not palpable. Correlate findings with history and obtain consultation as needed.

Prostatic carcinoma is the third leading cause of cancer death in men more than 55 years of age. Workers exposed to cadmium oxide are suspected of being at increased risk for developing prostatic carcinoma.

D. Technique. With gloved hand and lubricated second finger, press pad of examining finger against anal orifice to relax sphincter. Gently insert tip into anal canal with volar aspect of finger moving anteriorly toward patient's umbilicus. Palpate the bulging, rounded, posterior surface of the prostate at the anterior rectal wall (Fig. 11–7). Locate the median sulcus and the lateral lobes. Gently proceed superiorly along median sulcus. Just superior to the prostate lie the seminal vesicles on either side of the midline. These are palpable only when diseased. Next, proceed inferiorly along median sulcus and palpate just inferior to prostate for the bulbourethral glands. Again, these structures are usually palpable only when diseased. Complete examination of anus (see Chap. 10) and test any stool for occult blood. If a specimen is needed in a patient with chronic prostatitis, firmly massage prostate from lateral margins to median sulcus and gently milk the urethra. The fluid should be examined microscopically for leukocytes. If acute tenderness is noted, do not proceed with massage; obtain urinalysis to be examined for large mucous shreds suggesting acute prostatitis.

E. Normal findings. The prostate is approximately 1 inch (2.5 cm) in length, protruding posteriorly one-third to three-fourths inch (1–2 cm) into rectum. Only the posterior surface is palpable. Note two lateral lobes and a median furrow or sulcus. The patient normally describes sensation of pressure during digital examination.° The gland may be enlarged in the geriatric client.

F. Clinical alterations

   1. Absence of median sulcus in prostate hypertrophy.°

   2. Acute tenderness and possibly asymmetry and enlargement in prostatitis.

   3. Firm irregular nodules and asymmetry suggest carcinoma.°

   4. Palpable seminal vesicles owing to vesiculitis.

   5. Palpable, tender bulbourethral glands suggest cowperitis.

VI. Chart

   A. External genitalia: Normal distribution of pubic hair; circumcised penis; no swelling, lesions, or discharge; testicles descended, no tenderness or masses.

   B. Prostate: firm, nontender.

   C. Inguinal lymph nodes: no tender or enlarged nodes.

   D. Hernia: no mass or bulge.

Assessment of the
Female Genitalia

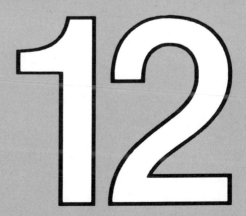

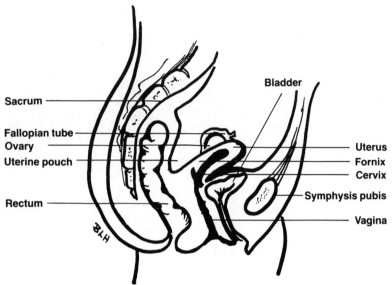

Figure 12–1. Cross section of the female genitalia.

I. Clinical considerations

A. A thorough knowledge of anatomy and physiology is necessary to accurately assess the female genitalia (Fig. 12–1).

B. The examination of the female genitalia includes inspection and palpation of the external genitalia, inspection of the visible internal reproductive structures by inserting a speculum, and palpation of the pelvic reproductive organs.

C. The client should be instructed not to douche or use tampons for 24 hours before the examination so as not to disturb the vaginal ecology.

D. The client may sit at a 45-degree angle during the examination of the external and internal genitalia and use a hand mirror to view her anatomic structures as they are being examined.

E. Equipment used for the internal examination (i.e., lubricant and speculum) should be warmed to normal body temperature.

F. The client should be encouraged to give verbal feedback throughout the examination so that the examiner is informed of any maneuvers that cause particular discomfort. This feedback will help maximize the client's cooperation and minimize her anxiety regarding the examination.

G. The pelvic examination is never a routine part of the physical examination of the child. Inspection and palpation of the external genitalia is all that should be included.

Menstrual patterns vary greatly among women. It is important, however, to know a client's normal cycle length to diagnose pregnancy, amenorrhea, or irregular bleeding problems. It is helpful to ask the client if she experiences dysmenorrhea (menstrual pain) because some women, especially young girls, frequently are disabled by this.

Premenstrual syndrome. A group of symptoms that occurs in a cyclic pattern prior to the onset of menses. These symptoms can range from breast bloating and tenderness to severe depression.

Menopause. The cessation of menses corresponding to declining levels of estrogen and ovarian function. Often menopause may be accompanied by symptoms of vasomotor instability such as hot flashes (rushes of heat sensation followed by rapid cooling producing diaphoresis) or ***formication*** (a sensation of bugs crawling on the skin).

Postmenopausal bleeding. Any bleeding that occurs after menopause. It is often the first sign of endometrial cancer.

Reproductive history is important to assess in relation to risk factors for cancer of the breast and uterus. The incidence of breast cancer is greater in women who are nulliparous or whose first pregnancy occurred after age 32. Endometrial cancer develops with greater frequency in nulliparous women.

Between 1940 and 1960 many women were treated for miscarriage with the estrogen diethylstilbestrol (DES). A number of gynecologic disorders have been documented in their offspring: adenocarcinoma of the vagina; noncancerous cellular anomalies such as vaginal adenosis and large cervical ectropions; and a number of anatomic anomalies such as hooded cervixes and small uteri.

II. Relevant history questions

A. Menstrual pattern.° Ask questions related to the following:

1. Age of menarche.

2. Date of last menstrual period (LMP).

3. Frequency of menstruation: time interval from the start of one menstrual period to the start of the next.

4. Character of menstrual flow such as length, amount, midcycle spotting, and clotting.

5. Associated phenomena such as menstrual pain, *premenstrual syndrome,* or irregular vaginal bleeding.

6. Age of *menopause* and accompanying vasomotor instability (hot flashes, headaches, palpitations, *formication*) and *postmenopausal bleeding.*

B. Reproductive history.° Ask questions related to the following:

1. Number of pregnancies: births, stillbirths, spontaneous abortions, therapeutic abortions, and age at time of first pregnancy.

2. Type of birth: vaginal delivery or cesarean section (cause).

3. Outcome: multiple pregnancies, prematurity, or low birth weight.

4. Complications such as medications, hemorrhage, or postpartum infection.

5. Infertility.

C. History of prenatal exposure to diethylstilbestrol.°

D. Exposure to sexually transmitted disease: ask questions related to the following:

1. Documented history of gonorrhea, syphilis, or genital herpes.

2. Recent exposure to a sexually transmitted disease.

3. Presence of chancre, foul discharge, or painful lesions.

Table 12–1. Characteristics of major types of **leukorrhea** (vaginal discharge)

	Normal		Cervical ectropion	Candidiasis	Trichomoniasis	Nonspecific vaginitis	Gonorrhea	Atrophic vaginitis
	Early cycle	Late cycle						
Color	Clear	White	Clear	White	Green or yellow	Gray or white	Yellow	Clear
Consistency	Elastic	Milky	Mucus	Dry cottage cheese	Bubbly liquid	Sticky liquid	Liquid	Liquid
Odor	None	None	None	None	Foul	Foul, fishy	Foul	None
Other symptoms	None	None or premenstrual itch	—	Itch; dyspareunia; symptoms increase with menses	Vulvar irritation	Slight itch	Dysuria; pelvic pain	Dryness; dyspareunia; vasomotor instability
Related factors	—	—	DES exposure	Birth control pills; diabetes mellitus; pregnancy; antibiotic therapy	Sexually transmitted	Sexually transmitted	Sexually transmitted	Menopause; low-estrogen birth control pills
Related physical examination findings	—	—	Ectropion	Erythema of vagina and vulva	Vaginal erythema; strawberry spots	—	Discharge from urethra or Skene's glands; pain on cervical motion	Thin, pale, dry mucosa

E. *Leukorrhea* (Table 12–1). Ask questions related to the following:

  1. Onset, quantity, color, consistency, odor, itching or irritation, and previous episodes.

  2. Predisposing factors such as oral contraceptives, recent antibiotic therapy, stress, exposure to sexually transmitted diseases, diabetes, or onset of menopause.

  3. Use of therapeutic modalities such as douches, tampons, or vaginal suppositories.

Papanicolaou (Pap) smear. Cytology specimens of superficial cells from the cervix.

Fibroid tumor. A fibrous, slow-growing benign tumor in the uterus. It may contraindicate the use of an intrauterine device (IUD).

Inorgasmic. Inability to achieve orgasm. This may be primary (never having experienced orgasm in the past) or secondary (experienced orgasm in past but not currently).

Dyspareunia. Painful intercourse. Dyspareunia may be due to vaginal dryness related to estrogen deficiency or candidiasis or caused by deep penetration of the pelvic organs by intercourse. The latter cause usually occurs in the presence of a pelvic infection, endometriosis, or an IUD.

Postcoital bleeding. Bleeding occurring immediately after intercourse. Postcoital bleeding can be attributed to a friable cervix from cervicitis or an early endometrial cancer.

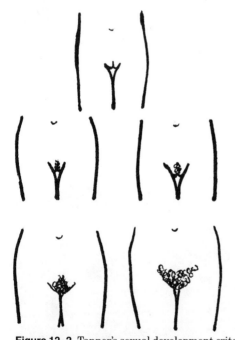

Figure 12–2. Tanner's sexual development criteria: pubic hair distribution.
1. Absent. 2. Sparse, lightly pigmented, straight; appears on inner border of labia.
3. Darker; increased amount; beginning to curl. 4. Coarse, curly; increased amount.
5. Adult distribution of inverted triangle with spread to thighs.

F. Prior gynecologic problems. Ask questions related to the following:

1. History of operations or endoscopic procedures.

2. Abnormal *Papanicolaou (Pap) smears.*

3. Ovarian cysts.

4. Endometriosis.

5. *Fibroid tumors.*

6. Carcinomas of the reproductive system.

G. Sexual function. Ask questions relating to the following:

1. Current sexual activity: type, multiple partners.

2. Satisfaction with sexual relations.

3. Associated phenomena such as inability to achieve orgasm (*inorgasmic*), *dyspareunia,* or *postcoital bleeding.*

4. Contraception

a. Method: oral contraceptive, diaphragm, intrauterine device, barrier methods, calendar methods, other.

b. Frequency of use and complications.

III. Inspection of the female genitalia. Position client so that she is relaxed in a lithotomy position with bladder empty. Buttocks should be positioned at the edge of the table. The client's upper torso may be at a 45-degree angle. Arms should be comfortably folded across her chest or down at her sides. The drape should be folded back across the lower abdomen to allow full visualization of the external genitalia. The examiner sits on a stool at the end of the table facing the client.

Instruct client to relax and breathe normally.

A. Inspect the external genitalia for the following development of secondary sexual characteristics.

1. **Note** distribution and presence and Tanner stage of pubic hair development. See Figure 12–2.

2. **Normal findings.** Varies with sexual maturity.

3. **Clinical alterations**

a. More than 10 percent of adult women in their late twenties have pubic hair that extends up the abdomen to the umbilicus.

b. Absent or scant distribution may indicate pituitary or adrenocortical dysfunction.

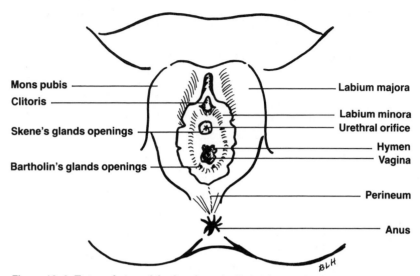

Figure 12-3. External view of the female genitalia (without pubic hair).

Genital herpes type II (herpes simplex). A sexually transmitted viral infection of the genital region. The virus generally is manifested by the presence of painful lesions occurring singly or in groups. These lesions may last from 1 to 3 weeks and are often precipitated by stressful events such as illness, menses, or nutritional deficiency states.

Nongonococcal urethritis (NGU). A bacterial infection of the urethra, most often caused by the organism chlamydia. NGU usually produces symptoms of dysuria.

B. Assess the mons pubis to determine the dermatologic condition of the pubic hair and underlying skin.

1. **Note** general hygiene and presence of lesions, *Phthirus pubis* (lice), or their eggs (nits).

2. **Normal findings.** Clean, coarse pubic hair; skin without lesions.

3. **Clinical alterations**

   a. Dirty-appearing hair shafts from pediculosis.

   b. Localized inflammation at the base of the hairshaft caused by folliculitis.

   c. Scaly epidermal plaques from psoriasis.

C. Inspect the vulva for genital lesions (Fig. 12–3).

1. **Note** cysts, warts, chancres, ulcerations, areas of hyperpigmentation.

2. **Normal findings.** Labia majora are hair-covered epidermal surfaces, labia minora are pink, glistening mucosal surfaces.

3. **Clinical alterations**

   a. Nontender, firm nodules of sebaceous cysts.

   b. Wartlike protrusions singly or in clusters from condyloma acuminatum or condyloma latum.

   c. Nontender chancre with a well-demarcated border from primary syphilis.

   d. Single or clustered tender ulcerations of **genital herpes type II.**

   e. Irregular, nontender hyperpigmented lesions related to carcinoma of the vulva.

D. Examine the clitoris.

1. **Note** size.

2. **Normal findings.** Round, pink tissue.

3. **Clinical alteration.** Enlargement in masculinizing conditions.

E. Inspect the urethral orifice.

1. **Note** erythema or purulent discharge.

2. **Normal findings.** Pink tissue without discharge.

3. **Clinical alterations**

   a. Purulent discharge of gonococcal urethritis.

   b. Thin, watery discharge of **nongonococcal urethritis** (NGU).

Cystocele. The prolapse of the bladder against the anterior vaginal wall. It is generally related to the weakening of vaginal and pelvic support by childbirth or operations.

Rectocele. The prolapse of the rectum against the posterior vaginal wall. It is generally related to the weakening of vaginal support by childbirth or operations.

Uterine prolapse. The protrusion of the lower uterine segment into the vagina. Most often this is due to the weakening of pelvic support by multiple child-births.

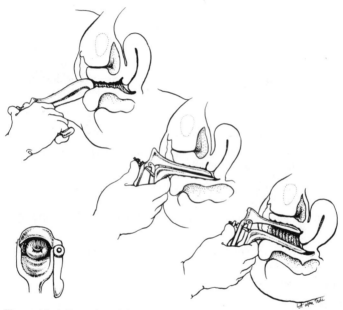

Figure 12–4. Insertion of the vaginal speculum. A. Blades held obliquely on entering the vagina. B. Blades rotated to the horizontal position as they pass the introitus. C. Blades separated by depressing thumbpiece and elevating handle. D. Normal parous cervix.

The speculum should not be lubricated because the jelly may affect the results of cultures or smears.

Estrogen deficiency syndrome. A condition by which the squamous epithelial tissue, which normally lines the vagina, becomes thin, friable, and subject to infection and trauma. These cellular changes are related to low estrogen levels that occur before menarche, during menopause, or with low-estrogen birth control pills.

Vaginal adenosis. Cellular changes that may be caused by prenatal exposure to DES. The condition may only be detected by colposcopy or the use of special staining procedures.

F. **Examine the vaginal orifice.**

1. **Note** presence of discharge, intact hymen, and bulging of vaginal tissue or cervix through the orifice.

2. **Normal findings.** Small amount of white discharge, intact hymen or hymenal remnants surrounding orifice; no bulging.

3. **Clinical alterations**

   a. Discharge secondary to vaginitis.

   b. Thin, pink membrane overlying the vaginal orifice from an imperforate hymen.

   c. Bulging of vaginal tissue through the orifice from a **cystocele** or **rectocele.**

   d. Appearance of the cervix in the vaginal orifice owing to **uterine prolapse.**

IV. **Speculum examination** (Fig. 12–4). **Position** client so that she maintains lithotomy position. **Instruct** client to be prepared to bear down when the speculum is inserted; then slowly inhale and exhale during the speculum examination. The client should inform the provider of any discomfort.

Technique: Insert index finger into vaginal orifice exerting pressure posteriorly. Insert forefinger in the same manner without removing index finger. Continuing downward pressure, obliquely insert the closed blades of an unlubricated speculum° with the opposite hand and slowly withdraw the fingers. Turn handle of speculum pointing downward and slide as far as possible into the vagina. Squeeze the handles of the speculum together and gently move the speculum to visualize the cervix. When the cervix is visualized, lock the speculum in place. To remove, gently withdraw the speculum so as not to pinch the cervix, collapse the handle, and continue to withdraw it from the vagina.

D. **Inspect the vaginal walls.**

1. **Note** surface for lesions and discharge.

2. **Normal findings.** Intact, pink, glistening rugate tissue.

3. **Clinical alterations**

   a. Pale friable tissue owing to **estrogen deficiency syndrome.**

   b. Discharge from vaginitis.

   c. Areas of nonsquamous epithelial cells on the vaginal walls caused by **vaginal adenosis.**

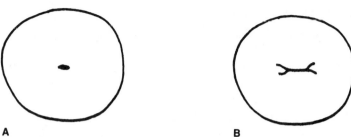

A   **B**
Figure 12–5. The cervix. A. Normal cervical os in a nulliparous woman. B. Normal cervical os in a parous woman.

Cervical ectropion. The presence of columnar cells on the cervix appearing as a red "erosion." Large ectropions may be present in women exposed to DES.

The specimens obtained form the Papanicolaou smear are interpreted as follows:

Class	Description
I	Negative
II	Atypical cells present; generally secondary to inflammation
III	Dysplasia present
IV	Carcinoma in situ
V	Carcinoma present

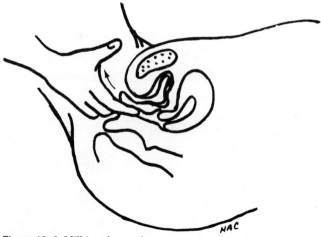

Figure 12–6. Milking the urethra.

E. Inspect the cervix (Fig. 12–5).

 1. **Note** color, shape of os, discharge, lesions, position, lacerations, presence of intrauterine device string; client discomfort.

 2. **Normal findings.** Pink surface with a central os. Os round or oval in nulliparous women; slit in parous women.

 3. **Clinical alterations**

   a. Inflammation and discharge from cervicitis.

   b. Eroded area on the cervix related to a **cervical ectropion.**

   c. Waxlike papules on cervix called nabothian cysts.

   d. Bluish hue of pregnancy.

   e. Red protrusion of a cervical polyp.

   f. Hard growth of carcinoma of the cervix.

F. Obtain a Papanicolaou (Pap) smear.°

 1. **Equipment**

   a. Glass slide

   b. Ayre's spatula

   c. Fixative

 2. **Instruction to client.** A slight pressure sensation may occur as cervix is scraped.

 3. **Technique**

   a. Press spatula tip against external cervical os.

   b. Rotate 360 degrees, maintaining equal pressure against cervix.

   c. Smear specimen on slide and immediately spray fixative.

V. Palpation of the internal and external genitalia. Position client so that she is in lithotomy position. She may either be supine or sitting at a 45-degree angle. Hands should be folded across the chest. Initially examiner sits at end of table and then stands at end of table for bimanual exam. **Instruct** client to be prepared to bear down when examiner's fingers are introduced into either the vagina or rectum. Client should inhale and exhale slowly throughout the examination. Client should inform examiner of any discomfort.

A. Assess paraurethral glands and urethra.

 1. **Technique.** Insert gloved index finger into the vagina while maintaining steady pressure upwards; remove the finger, milking the urethra (Fig. 12–6).

 2. **Note** discharge from the urethra, paraurethral glands, or tenderness.

 3. **Clinical alteration.** Purulent discharge from paraurethral glands related to gonococcal urethritis.

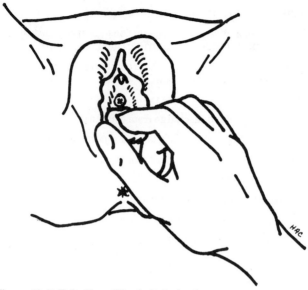

Figure 12–7. Palpation of Bartholin's glands.

Bartholin's cyst. Swelling of Bartholin's gland. Swelling may be a chronic problem owing to the accumulation of clear fluid. If the swollen gland becomes painful, it is called Bartholin's abscess.

B. **Assess Bartholin's glands.**

1. **Technique.** Insert index finger into vagina with thumb remaining outside on the posterior portion of the labia majora. Press thumb and index finger together to assess the gland; then do the same on the opposite side (Fig. 12–7).

2. **Note** bulging, tenderness, and discharge.

3. **Normal findings.** No enlargement, tenderness, or discharge.

4. **Clinical alteration.** Bulging of gland from a *Bartholin's cyst* or abscess.

C. **Assess vaginal wall support.**

1. **Instruction to client.** Bear down.

2. **Technique.** Separate the vaginal orifice with the thumb and index finger.

3. **Note** bulging of anterior or posterior vaginal wall.

4. **Normal findings.** None.

5. **Clinical alteration.** Visible bulging of anterior or posterior vaginal walls related to a cystocele or rectocele.

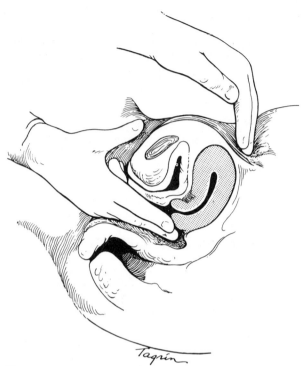

Figure 12–8. Bimanual abdominovaginal palpation of the uterus.

Ovarian cysts may occur in women of all ages. They arise from the collection of fluid or debris within a sac formed from different layers of cells within the ovary. Although most cysts are benign, some can lead to a malignancy if not treated.

Ectopic pregnancy. The implantation of a fertilized ovum within the fallopian tube causing pain and swelling of the tube. If not immediately treated, the tube can rupture, causing a life-threatening situation.

The ovaries are the third most common site of malignancy in the female reproductive tract. Ovarian cancer occurs most often after menopause; a high mortality is associated with it.

Endometriosis. The presence of endometrial tissue outside the uterus. It is often found on the ovary and adjacent structures in the pelvic cavity. At menstruation these ectopic sites bleed as do normal endometrium, thus causing increased pain and flow.

D. Bimanually assess the uterus.

1. **Technique.** Insert first and second fingers into the vagina with the palmar surface anteriorly. Apply firm pressure on the posterior surface of the cervix to ballot the uterus into the lower abdomen. With the other hand, press firmly on the abdomen with the palmar surface (Fig. 12–8). Assess the uterus with the abdominal hand.

2. **Note** size, consistency, tenderness, mobility, and masses.

3. **Normal findings.** Smooth, firm surface, mobile, without tenderness or masses.

4. **Clinical alterations**

   a. Soft; enlargement from an intrauterine pregnancy.

   b. Tenderness of uterus and fallopian tubes especially with motion of the lower uterine segment related to pelvic inflammatory disease.

   c. Specific tenderness of the posterior surface of the uterus because of endometriosis.

   d. Irregular, firm uterus related to fibroids.

   e. Irregular, rockhard uterus related to cancer.

E. Bimanually assess the ovaries and fallopian tubes.

1. **Instructions to client.** A fleeting sensation of discomfort may be felt when the ovaries are examined.

2. **Technique.** Move the internal first and second fingers to the lateral fornix. Move the abdominal hand to the lower abdominal quadrant on the same side as the internal hand. Move the abdominal hand slowly toward the fornix to move the ovary against the internal hand for assessment. Repeat on opposite side.

3. **Note** size, consistency, masses, and tenderness.

4. **Normal findings.** Mobile, firm, ovoid structure.

5. **Clinical alterations**

   a. Swelling on ovary owing to the presence of an ovarian cyst.°

   b. Tender mass in the fallopian tube from an ***ectopic pregnancy.***

   c. Hard ovarian mass from cancer of the ovary.°

   d. Tenderness of ovary, fallopian tubes, or both owing to ***endometriosis.***

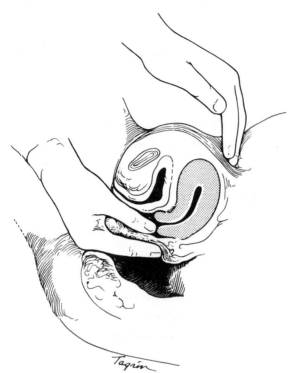

Figure 12–9. Bidigital rectovaginal examination.

F. **Assess the posterior uterus and supporting structures rectova-ginally.**

1. **Instructions to client.** Bear down when the finger is inserted into the rectum; then relax and continue to inhale and exhale slowly. Describe any discomfort.

2. **Technique.** Remove the internal hand from the vagina, change gloves, lubricate the first finger, and insert it into the rectum while the thumb of the same hand is being reintroduced into the vagina (Fig. 12–9). Insert the fingers as far as possible. With the other hand on the abdomen, push the uterus as posteriorly as possible. The internal fingers should be able to assess the poste-rior surface of the uterus. Complete examination of the anus (see Chapter 10).

3. **Note** size, consistency, tenderness, mobility, and masses.

4. **Normal findings.** Smooth, mobile uterus without masses or ten-derness.

5. **Clinical alterations**

   a. Tenderness on the uterosacral ligament or severe uterine retroversion owing to endometriosis.

   b. Smooth, irregular uterus from fibroids.

   c. Rockhard, fixed uterus because of uterine cancer.

VI. **Chart.**

A. **External genitalia:** normal distribution of pubic hair; no lesions or growths; all structures present without deformities.

B. **Bartholin's gland, urethra:** no masses or discharge.

C. **Vagina:** pink, rugate without bulging; no discharge apparent.

D. **Cervix:** pink; no lesions apparent.

E. **Uterus:** anterior; firm without enlargement, tenderness, or masses.

F. **Adnexae:** ovaries palpated without tenderness or masses.

Assessment of the Musculoskeletal System

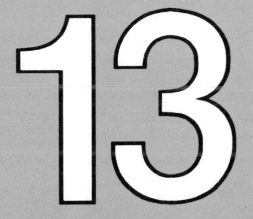

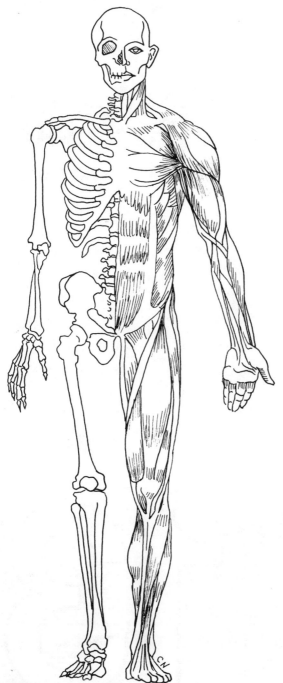

Figure 13–1. The musculoskeletal anatomy (Anterior view).

I. Clinical considerations

A. A thorough knowledge of the anatomy of the musculoskeletal system is essential (Fig. 13–1).

B. Assessment of the musculoskeletal system includes inspection, palpation, percussion, and auscultation.

C. Symmetry should be observed during both the general and local examinations.

D. The examination begins with inspection of the client as soon as he or she enters the room.

E. The client must disrobe for a thorough examination.

F. If injury has occurred or if pain is present in a joint, the following must be examined:

 1. The joints proximally and distally.

 2. Neurologic function including motor strength, deep tendon reflexes, and sensation.

 3. Peripheral vascular function.

 4. Adjacent soft tissue.

 5. Structures or organs supplied by the same nerves.

G. Any discomfort elicited during the examination should be reported by the client.

Active range of motion. The client moves his or her own joints.

Passive range of motion. The examiner moves the joint while the client keeps his or her muscles relaxed.

Joint stability is assessed by stressing the stabilizing ligaments.

Motor strength should be graded on a scale of 0 to 5. (See Chap. 14,**VII.J.**)

Integrated function. Tests the coordination of different parts of the musculo-skeletal system and between the musculoskeletal and neurologic systems. It includes testing of the deep tendon reflexes and perception of touch and pain.

Bone pain, unless it is due to a fracture or a bruise, is deep and boring, often intense, not related to movement, often worse at night keeping the client awake, and possibly intensified by weight bearing.
Joint pain is generally localized or proximate to a joint. Movement and weight bearing generally aggravate the pain, and rest usually relieves it. The onset may be gradual or sudden and there may be migration from joint to joint.
Muscle pain often results from unusual, prolonged, or excessive exercise. It generally subsides with rest. If the muscle or tendon has been torn, the pain may be progressive during the inflammatory process. Tendon inflammation gives rise to intense localized pain, which may be aggravated by movement and relieved by rest.
Referred pain results from compression of a nerve that supplies the painful area, or it may be from a disease of a structure that is served by the same nerve as the painful area.

Obtaining occupational history aids the examiner in assessing the relationship between the work environment and the musculoskeletal system. Some muscu-loskeletal problems occur more frequently in clients of certain occupations. This information helps in assessing a cause but should not negate obtaining a thorough history. The information from an occupational history helps the ex-aminer judge the client's ability to perform certain tasks as well as his or her ability to return to work after injury.

Recreational history is obtained to help diagnose the cause of a complaint. Cer-tain recreational activities predispose the client to musculoskeletal complaints.

General survey. Includes observation of posture, gait, and ordinary physical activities.

Equipment such as canes, crutches, and braces that the client is currently us-ing or has used should be noted. The use of such aids clues the examiner to the client's actual or perceived weakness, instability, or pain.

H. There are two parts to assessment of the musculoskeletal system: the general overview and the regional examinations, which include the systematic, bilateral examination of the joints for alignment, *active* and *passive range of motion,* structural abnormalities, immobility, joint stability,° tenderness, inflammation, motor strength,° and *integrated function.*

I. There are many common clinical alterations that can affect each joint. Sports injuries are common during adolescence and young adulthood; arthritis is common in the geriatric client.

J. Range of motion techniques are best performed after the examiner demonstrates the maneuver to the client.

II. Relevant history questions

A. Pain.° Ask questions related to the following:

1. Onset, quantity, quality, location, duration, timing, radiation, and history of musculoskeletal problems.

2. Relationship to movement.

3. Predisposing factors such as unusual or prolonged activity.

4. Factors related to injury (such as the mechanism of injury, force, the duration of force, time of injury, onset of pain, disability, swelling, and discoloration) and history of previous injury.

5. Associated signs and symptoms such as deformity, swelling, heat, erythema, weakness, limitation of motion, stiffness, paresthesias, or constitutional symptoms.

6. Aggravating or alleviating factors such as position, supports, and medications.

B. Occupational history.° Ask questions related to present and past occupations, specific activities performed, others at work with same complaint.

C. Recreational history.° Ask questions related to specific sports and hobbies.

D. Functional assessment. Ask questions related to activities of daily living the client is able to perform and adjustments or aids being used.

III. Examination of the musculoskeletal system: Conduct the *general survey.*

A. Technique. Observe client as he or she enters the room, moves about the room, disrobes, and moves on and off the examining table. Observe posture from the front, back, and sides.

B. Note ease of movement, posture, gait, and use of any equipment.°

C. Normal findings. Movement smooth; straight alignment of the trunk; symmetry of shoulders, pelvis, scapulae, and buttock creases; equal stride length; and symmetry of arm swing.

Temporomandibular joint. The articulation between the mandible and the skull. It should be assessed in the presence of ear and jaw pain.

The patient may have associated symptoms of locking the jaw or grating or popping when chewing or talking.

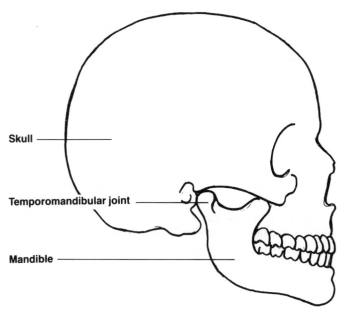

Skull

Temporomandibular joint

Mandible

Figure 13–2. Anatomic location of the temporomandibular joint.

Crepitation. A grating sound or palpable sensation owing to roughness of the articular surfaces.

Range of motion: the client should be able to open his or her mouth to a distance of three finger breadths (2 inches).

Trismus. Inability to open mouth.

D. **Clinical alterations**

1. Asymmetry owing to kyphosis, scoliosis, or lordosis.

2. Instability from cerebellar disease, peripheral neuropathy, cerebrovascular accident, or pain.

IV. **Examination of the *temporomandibular joint*°** (Fig. 13–2). **Position** client so that he or she is sitting up facing the examiner.

A. **Inspect the temporomandibular joint.**

1. **Technique.** Systematically observe the temporomandibular joint and the posture of the neck.

2. **Note** color, alignment, and bony deformities.

3. **Normal findings.** Symmetric appearance, no deformities.

4. **Clinical alteration.** Protrusion of the mandible from dislocation.

B. **Palpate the temporomandibular joint.**

1. **Technique.** Palpate each joint anterior to the tragus of the ear.

2. **Note** heat, swelling, effusion, bony enlargement, bogginess, and tenderness.

3. **Normal findings.** Nontender, without enlargements.

4. **Clinical alteration.** Tenderness owing to rheumatoid arthritis or temporomandibular joint syndrome.

C. **Evaluate the temporomandibular joint for range of motion and for tenderness and *crepitation* when client demonstrates range of motion.**

1. **Instructions to client.** Open and close your mouth widely when asked to do so.

2. **Technique.** Palpate each temporomandibular joint as the client opens and closes his mouth.

3. **Alternate technique.** Place finger in acoustic meatus, pull forward as client opens and closes mouth.

4. **Note** tenderness, crepitation, clicking, and limitation of motion.°

5. **Normal findings.** Smooth movement of the mandible.

6. **Clinical alterations**

a. Crepitus associated with rheumatoid arthritis.

b. Clicking owing to displaced cartilage.

c. *Trismus* from muscle spasm.

D. **Common clinical alterations.** See **XVI.**

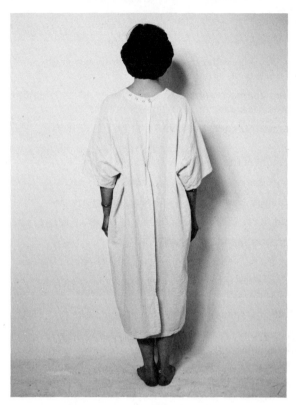

Figure 13–3. Assessment of the cervical spine.

The cervical spine consists of seven cervical vertebrae (C-1 through C-7). C-1 and C-2 provide motion; C-3 through the first thoracic vertebrae (T-1) provide support (most radiologic abnormalities are seen here).

The most prominent spinous process when flexing the neck is usually C-7 but may be T-1.

Ankylosing spondylosis. Immobility or fixation of a joint caused by degeneration of the vertebrae and their disks.

Whiplash. Injury caused by sudden and forceful hyperextension of the cervical spine, with flexion recoil. Whiplash often occurs to persons riding in a car that is struck from behind. Tenderness is often associated with headache, blurring of vision, and a soft crepitus.

V. **Examination of the cervical spine.**° **Position** client so that he or she is sitting or standing in front of the examiner with upper back area exposed (Fig. 13–3).

A. Inspect the cervical spine.

1. **Technique.** Systematically inspect the cervical spine from the front, sides, and back.

2. **Note** prominences,° color, bony deformities, and alignment.

3. **Normal findings.** Concave posture; straight spinal alignment.

4. **Clinical alteration.** Lateral deviation from torticollis or pain.

B. Palpate the cervical spine.

1. **Instructions to client.** Describe any tenderness.

2. **Technique.** Palpate each spinous process.

3. **Note** heat, swelling, deformities, and tenderness.

4. **Normal findings.** Nontender; no deformities.

5. **Clinical alterations**

   a. Tenderness from ***ankylosing spondylosis.***

   b. Tenderness in posterior cervical muscles owing to nuchal headache.

C. Percuss the cervical spine.

1. **Equipment.** Rubber hammer.

2. **Technique.** Percuss the spinous processes with the hand or rubber hammer.

3. **Note** tenderness.

4. **Normal findings.** Nontender.

5. **Clinical alteration.** Tenderness from a disorder in the vertebrae or a cervical ***whiplash*** injury.

Table 13–1. Range of motion of the neck

Motion	Range (degrees)
Flexion	45
Extension	45
Lateral bending	45
Rotation	70

Paravertebral muscles are composed of three layers of muscles. Only the superficial layer, the sacrospinal system, is palpable.

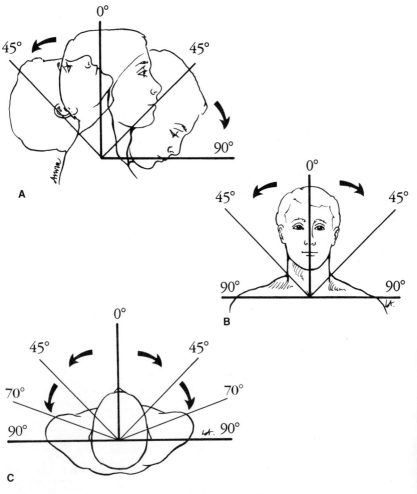

Figure 13–4. Passive range of motion of the neck: A. Flexion and extension. B. Lateral bending. C. Rotation.

D. **Evaluate the cervical spine for range of motion and tenderness, crepitation, or muscle spasm when client demonstrates range of motion** (Table 13–1).

  1. **Instructions to client.** Close your mouth and be prepared to maneuver head as instructed. Describe any discomfort.

  2. **Technique.** Palpate the neck as the client flexes chin to chest, rotates chin to each shoulder, laterally bends each ear to corresponding shoulder, and extends head backward. Palpate the paravertebral muscles° with the flat of the hand.

  3. **Note** tenderness, crepitation, limitation of motion, and muscle spasm.

  4. **Normal findings.** Smooth, full range of motion (Fig. 13–4); no tenderness.

  5. **Clinical alterations**

     a. Stiff neck associated with meningitis or muscle spasm.

     b. Limitation on extension and lateral bending owing to herniation of a cervical disk.

     c. Pain and crepitus seen in traumatic fracture.

Meningial signs are checked if inflammation of the meninges is suspected. Meningial signs are:

1. Nuchal rigidity. Client unable to flex chin on chest.

2. Spinal rigidity. Client has limited movement of the spine, producing rigid hyperextension.

Often one shoulder is higher.

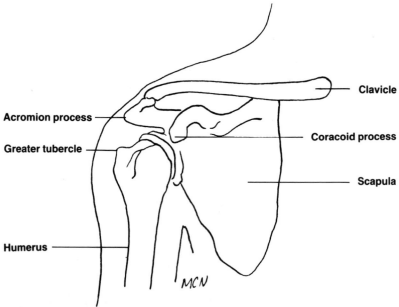

Figure 13–5. Right shoulder joint.

E. **Thoroughly examine the temporomandibular joint, lower jaw, teeth, thyroid gland, and scalp if client has neck pain and the history is suggestive.**

F. **Check *meningial signs* if client has neck pain.**

G. **Common clinical alterations.** See **XVI.**

VI. **Examination of the shoulder** (Fig. 13–5). **Position** client so that he or she is seated with shoulders exposed.

A. **Inspect the shoulders.**

   1. **Technique.** Systematically inspect the shoulders from the front, sides, back, and above.

   2. **Note** color, swelling, deformities, alignment, and muscular atrophy.

   3. **Normal findings.** Intact, smooth, and regular; bilaterally symmetric.°

   4. **Clinical alterations**

      a. Muscle atrophy from nerve compression.

      b. Swelling from arthritis.

      c. Deformity from dislocation of the shoulder.

B. **Inspect the scapulae from the back.**

   1. **Position.** Client flexes arms forward 90 degrees.

   2. **Technique.** The examiner creates resistance by pushing downward on the client's flexed arms. The client resists by pushing upward.

   3. **Normal findings.** Bilaterally symmetric with borders held firm to chest wall.

   4. **Clinical alterations**

      a. Winging of the scapulae often indicates weakness of the serratus anterior muscles.

      b. Asymmetric scapulae owing to scoliosis.

The tendons of the supraspinatus, infraspinatus, and teres minor insert on the greater tuberosity forming the rotator cuff. The tendon of the subscapularis, also part of the rotator cuff, inserts on the lesser tuberosity. The biceps brachii tendon is in the biceps groove.

Supraspinatus tendinitis. Deposit of calcium in the supraspinatus tendon producing acute inflammation.

Table 13–2. Range of motion of the shoulder

Motion	Range (degrees)
Forward flexion	180
Extension	45
Abduction	180
Adduction	90
Inward rotation	90
Outward rotation	90

C. **Palpate the shoulder.**

1. **Instructions to client.** Describe any tenderness.

2. **Technique.** Palpate the sternoclavicular joint, along the clavicle, the acromioclavicular joint, and the scapular spine. Palpate the greater and lesser tuberosity of the humerus and the biceps groove° between the greater and lesser tuberosity. Next, palpate the subdeltoid bursa.

3. **Note** heat, swelling, bony enlargement, tenderness, and muscular atrophy.

4. **Normal findings.** Nontender, smooth, and regular; bilaterally symmetric.

5. **Clinical alterations**

   a. Tenderness owing to tendinitis of the biceps.

   b. Localized tenderness at the acromial tip from **supraspinatus tendinitis.**

   c. Atrophy of the cuff muscles suggestive of tear of rotator cuff.

D. **Examine the shoulder for range of motion and for tenderness and crepitation when client demonstrates range of motion** (Table 13–2).

1. **Instructions to client.** Be prepared to maneuver shoulder as instructed.

2. **Technique.** Palpate the shoulder by cupping hand over the shoulder as the client adducts arm across his or her body, abducts arm straight out to the side, flexes arm straight forward, extends arm backward, and internally and externally rotates shoulder.

3. **Note** tenderness, crepitation, limitation of motion.

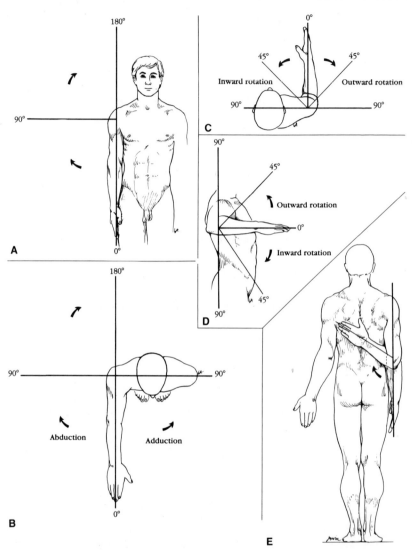

Figure 13–6. Passive range of motion of the shoulder. A. Elevation. B. Abduction-adduction. C. Rotation with arm at side. D. Rotation in 90° elevation and 90° abduction. E. Internal rotation posteriorly.

Pain in the shoulder may be referred from the heart, lungs, spine, diaphragm, or vasculature.

4. **Normal findings.** Smooth, full range of motion (Fig. 13–6); no tenderness or crepitation.

5. **Clinical alteration.** Pain and crepitus on range of motion commonly associated with supraspinatus tendinitis, rotator cuff tear, arthritis, or bursitis.

E. **Thoroughly examine the cervical spine and elbow if client has shoulder pain.**

F. **Examine the heart, lungs, and abdomen if pain is present and if the history is appropriate.**°

G. **Common clinical alterations.** See section **XVI.**

In examining the elbow, it is important to correlate the findings with an occupational history as well as a recreational history.

Carrying angle. The angle formed by the upper and lower arm when the elbow is observed from the front with the forearm in full extension and supination.

Olecranon bursitis is common in miners and students. The swelling is fluctuant.

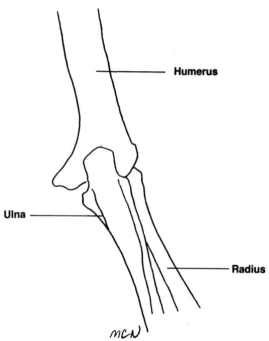

Figure 13–7. Right elbow joint.

Tennis elbow. A condition causing pain in the lateral epicondyle region and extensor muscle origin of the elbow. It is often present in tennis players, with the pain related to repetitive pronation and supination of the forearm.

VII. Examination of the elbow° (Fig. 13–7). **Position** client so that he or she is standing with elbows exposed and arms in anatomic position.

A. **Inspect the elbow.**

1. **Technique.** Systematically inspect the extensor and flexor surface of the elbow.

2. **Note** color, swelling, bony deformities, atrophy, and **carrying angle.**

3. **Normal findings.** Smooth and regular; valgus angulation of 5 degrees in men, 10 to 15 degrees in women.

4. **Clinical alterations**

   a. Swelling often from olecranon bursitis° or arthritis.

   b. Deformity from dislocation of the elbow.

B. **Palpate the elbow.**

1. **Instructions to client.** Describe any tenderness.

2. **Technique.** Palpate the extensor and flexor surfaces. Palpate the biceps tendon in the cubital fossa and the area of the olecranon bursa overlying the olecranon process of the ulna. Palpate the groove on either side of the olecranon. Palpate the medial and lateral epicondyle of the humerus and the radial head.

3. **Note** heat, swelling, bony enlargement, tenderness, atrophy, and nodules.

4. **Normal findings.** Nontender; smooth and regular without nodules; decreased muscle in the aged client.

5. **Clinical alterations**

   a. Tenderness over the lateral epicondyle from **tennis elbow.**

   b. Rheumatoid nodules common in the olecranon bursa and distally.

   c. Tenderness owing to fractures.

Table 13–3. Range of motion of the elbow

Motion	Range (degrees)
Flexion	160
Supination	90
Pronation	90

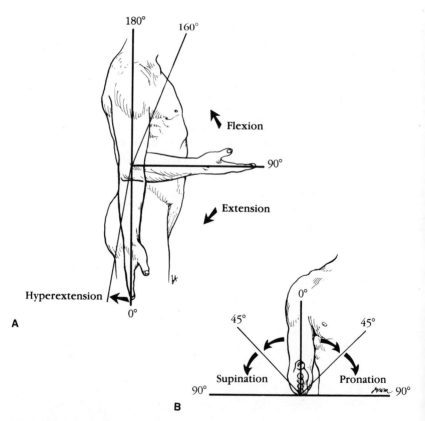

Figure 13–8. Passive range of motion of the elbow. A. Flexion and extension. B. Forearm (elbow and wrist).

C. **Evaluate the elbow for range of motion and tenderness and crepitation when client demonstrates range of motion** (Table 13–3).

1. **Instructions to client.** Be prepared to perform various maneuvers when asked.

2. **Technique.** The client's elbow is placed into the examiner's palm as the client flexes elbow by touching hand to shoulder. He or she then extends elbow by straightening arm. Palpate the elbow in the same manner as the client flexes elbow to 90 degrees. The examiner next holds the upper arm stationary as the client supinates the forearm by turning the palms up and pronates by turning the palms down.

3. **Note** tenderness, crepitation, and limitation of motion.

4. **Normal findings.** Full, smooth range of motion (Fig. 13–8); nontender; no crepitation.

5. **Clinical alterations**

   a. Pain on range of motion often from rheumatoid arthritis.

   b. Crepitus with minimal pain on range of motion associated with osteoarthritis.

D. **Assess the client's function** (i.e., can the patient wash his or her face, button collar?).

E. **Thoroughly examine the cervical spine, shoulder, and wrist if client has elbow pain.**

F. **Common clinical alterations.** See **XVI.**

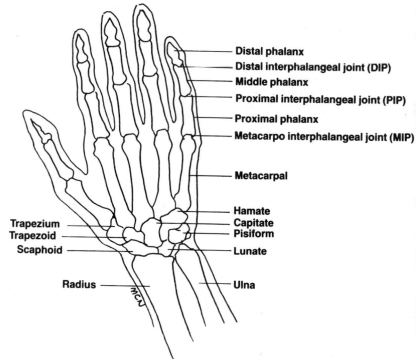

Figure 13–9. Bones of the hand and wrist.

Anatomical snuff-box. A triangular area at the base of the thumb bounded by the extensor pollicis longus on the ulnar aspect and by the extensor pollicis brevis on the radial aspect.

The scaphoid and lunate bones are the most frequently affected in traumatic injuries. The most common area of fracture is at the wrist, and subsequent ischemic necrosis may result.

Carpal tunnel syndrome. Compression of the medial nerve. Symptoms are numbness and tingling, particularly at night. Light percussion may reproduce a tingling sensation and is a positive Tinel's sign. Pain may be reproduced by flexion of the wrist for 60 seconds. The palms are generally dry in clients with carpal tunnel syndrome.

Ganglion. A cystic, generally painless nodule located along the tendon sheaths commonly found on the dorsums of the hand and wrist. Flexion of the wrist accentuates a ganglion.

VIII. **Examination of the wrist** (Fig. 13–9). **Position** client so that he or she is seated.

A. **Inspect the wrist.**

1. **Technique.** Systematically inspect the volar and dorsal aspects of the wrist.

2. **Note** color, swelling, fluid in the joint, bony enlargement, and deformities.

3. **Normal findings.** Smooth; without swelling or deformities.

4. **Clinical alterations**

a. Swelling on dorsum from a ganglion.

b. Enlarged bones owing to osteophytosis.

B. **Palpate the volar and dorsal aspects of the wrist.**

1. **Instructions to client.** Describe any tenderness.

2. **Technique.** Palpate the ulnar head, ulnar styloid process, and radial styloid process. The scaphoid, just distal to the styloid process, is palpated in the **anatomical snuff-box** by having the client's thumb in extension and abduction. The lunate is palpated immediately distal to the dorsal tubercle of the radius. The pisiform is next palpated just distal to the ulnar styloid process. Conclude by palpating the extensor and flexor tendons.

3. **Note** heat, swelling, deformities, bony enlargements, and tenderness.

4. **Normal findings.** Smooth; nontender.

5. **Clinical alterations**°

a. Pain, numbness, and tingling of the hand owing to **carpal tunnel syndrome.**

b. Tender, swelling in the anatomist's snuff-box from acute nonsuppurative tenosynovitis.

c. Nontender swelling from a **ganglion.**

Table 13–4. Range of motion of the wrist

Motion	Range (degrees)
Radial deviation	25
Ulnar deviation	25
Flexion	45
Extension	45

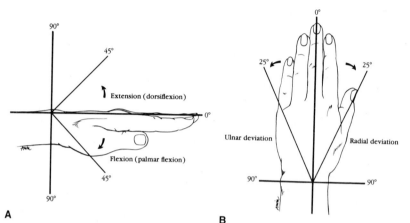

Figure 13–10. Passive range of motion of the wrist. A. Flexion and extension. B. Lateral deviation.

Sensory distribution of the hand is as follows:

1. Median nerve: volar side of thumb, index and middle fingers, and radial half of ring finger from tip to wrist; dorsal side of index and middle fingers from tip to proximal interphalangeal joints (PIP).

2. Radial nerve: dorsum of thumb to the tip; dorsum of index and middle fingers from the proximal interphalangeal joint (PIP) to wrist.

3. Ulnar nerve: dorsal and volar sides of the ulnar half of the ring finger and the entire little finger from tip to wrist.

C. **Evaluate the wrist for range of motion and tenderness and crepitation when client demonstrates range of motion** (Table 13–4).

1. **Instructions to client.** Be prepared to maneuver wrist as asked.

2. **Technique.** The client's wrist should be placed in the examiner's palm and the client asked to flex wrist by bending it down and extending it. The client should be asked to deviate the ulnar bone by turning the hand toward the little finger while the examiner holds the forearm stationary. Deviate the radial bone toward the thumb in a similar fashion.

3. **Note** tenderness, crepitation, and limitation of motion.

4. **Normal findings.** Full, smooth range of motion (Fig. 13–10); nontender; no crepitation.

5. **Clinical alterations**

    a. Decreased motor function from carpal tunnel syndrome.

    b. Pain and crepitus owing to tenosynovitis.

D. **Thoroughly examine the cervical spine, shoulders, arm, elbow, and hand if wrist pain is present or injury has occurred.**

E. **Assess sensory distribution.**°

F. **Common clinical alterations.** See **XVI.**

Normal posture of the hand is with the wrist slightly extended. The metacarpophalangeal and interphalangeal joints are slightly flexed, and the thumb rests on the index and middle fingers.

Small muscle atrophy is common in the geriatric client. Atrophy of the dorsal muscle leaves grooves and concavities. There may be flattening of the thenar and hypothenar eminences.

Heberden's nodes. Small, hard, generally painless nodules that occur over the dorsolateral aspect of the distal interphalangeal joints. They are often associated with trauma or osteoarthritis.

Bouchard's nodes. Similar to but less common than Heberden's nodes and are found on the proximal interphalangeal joints.

Dupuytren's contracture. Thickened, fibrotic cord between the palm and finger, forcing the affected finger into partial flexion.

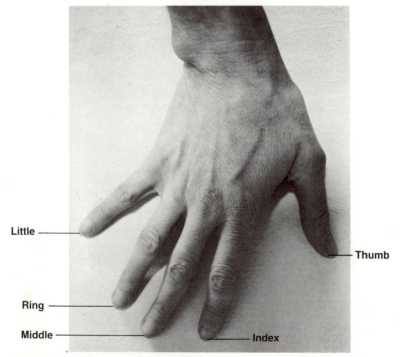

Figure 13–11. Dorsal aspect of the right hand.

IX. Examination of the hand and fingers (see Fig. 13–9). **Position** client so that he or she is seated.

   A. Inspect the hand and fingers.

   1. **Technique.** Systematically inspect the dorsal and palmar surfaces.

   2. **Note** color, swelling, symmetry, posture,° deformities, skeletal enlargement, muscular atrophy, and nodes.

   3. **Normal findings.** Smooth, bilaterally symmetric, without swelling or deformities; small muscle atrophy° in the geriatric client.

   4. **Clinical alterations**

      a. Swelling of joints and ulnar deviation from chronic rheumatoid arthritis.

      b. Radial deviation of the distal phalynx and *Heberden's nodes* or *Bouchard's nodes.*

      c. Flexion contracture of the fingers from *Dupuytren's contracture.*

      d. Tophi associated with gouty arthritis.

   B. Palpate the dorsal and palmer surfaces of the hand and fingers (Fig. 13–11).

   1. **Instructions to client.** Describe any tenderness.

   2. **Technique.** Palpate each metacarpophalangeal and interphalangeal joint, both in the dorsoventral plane and the mediolateral direction. Compress each metacarpophalangeal joint by placing thumb on dorsal surface, fingers in palmar surface. Progress along each metacarpal on both dorsal and palmer surfaces.

   3. **Note** heat or coldness, moisture, dryness, swelling, deformities, tenderness, muscular atrophy, nodes, bony enlargement, bogginess, thickening, and palpable flexor tendons.

   4. **Normal findings.** Smooth, nontender; small muscle atrophy in the elderly client.

   5. **Clinical alterations**

      a. Nodes owing to osteoarthritis.

      b. Coldness and increased moisture may indicate excess sympathetic activity.

      c. Dryness may indicate damage to a nerve supplying the area.

      d. Tenderness and swelling from rheumatoid arthritis or osteoarthritis.

Table 13–5. Range of motion of the finger

Motion	Range (degrees)
Metacarp phalangeal joint	
Flexion	90
Hyperextension	30
Extension	45
Proximal interphalangeal: flexion	120
Distal interphalangeal joint	
Flexion	80
Hyperextension	10
Thumb abduction: flexion	90
Interphalangeal joint: flexion	80
Metacarpophalangeal joint: flexion	50
Carpometacarpal joint: flexion	15
Opposition: flexion	Thumb flexes to the base of the little finger

C. **Evaluate hand for range of motion and tenderness and crepitation when client demonstrates range of motion** (Table 13–5).

   1. **Instructions to client.** Be prepared to maneuver hand as instructed.

   2. **Technique.** Assess hand as the client performs the following maneuvers:

      a. Flexes fingers, making a fist; extends fingers by straightening them out.

      b. Abducts and adducts fingers by spreading and closing them.

      c. Abducts thumb and demonstrates opposition by touching tip of thumb to fifth metacarpophalangeal joint.

      d. Flexes the thumb by folding it inward toward the palmar surface and extends it by straightening it.

   3. **Note** tenderness, crepitation, and limitation of motion.

   4. **Normal findings.** Symmetric response; smooth movement, full range of motion.

   5. **Clinical alteration.** Pain and decreased range of motion associated with rheumatoid arthritis, osteoarthritis, or gouty arthritis.

D. **Thoroughly examine the cervical spine, shoulders, elbow, and wrist if hand pain is present.**

E. **Common clinical alterations.** See **XVI.**

The actual hip joint is inaccessible to examination. Adjacent structures must be carefully examined.

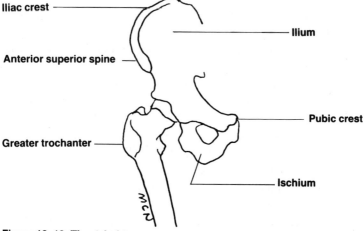

Figure 13–12. The right hip.

The trochanteric bursa overlies the greater trochanter.

The sciatic nerve lies halfway between the ischial tuberosity and the greater trochanter.

X. Examination of the hip (Fig. 13–12).° **Position** client so that he or she is standing. The examiner is behind.

A. **Inspect the hip posteriorly.**

    1. **Technique.** Observe the iliac spines, spinal curvature, level of the posterior superior iliac crest, level of the gluteal folds, posture of the legs, and position of the feet as they contact the ground. Observe gait.

    2. **Note** asymmetry in level of landmarks, exaggerated spinal curvatures, scoliosis, flexed or hyperextended leg joints, and portion of sole in contact with ground.

    3. **Normal findings.** Bilaterally symmetric; entire sole in contact with ground.

    4. **Clinical alterations**

        a. Waddling gait seen in bilateral hip dislocation.

        b. Swinging of leg often from ankylosis.

B. **Inspect the hip anteriorly.**

    1. **Position.** Client is supine.

    2. **Technique.** Systematically inspect the hip and groin area.

    3. **Note** color, swelling, deformity, and muscular atrophy.

    4. **Normal findings.** Hips bilaterally symmetric; hip in full extension.

    5. **Clinical alterations.** See **X.A.4.**

C. **Palpate the hip.**

    1. **Instructions to client.** Describe any tenderness.

    2. **Technique.** Palpate the buttocks, deep inguinal area, and femoral triangle for lymph nodes and pulsation of the femoral artery. Then proceed laterally to the area of the greater trochanter.° Palpate the accessible bony points including the iliac crests with their spines, pubic crests and tubercles, greater trochanters, and the ischiatic tuberosities. Palpate the sciatic nerve° through the gluteus maximus with the hip flexed.

    3. **Note** heat, swelling, and tenderness.

    4. **Normal findings.** Nontender; bilaterally symmetric.

    5. **Clinical alterations**

        a. Tenderness owing to compression of the sciatic nerve.

        b. Palpable swelling owing to osteoarthritis.

Table 13–6. Range of motion of the hip

Motion	Range (degrees)
Internal rotation	45
External rotation	45
Abduction	45
Adduction	30
Rotation with the knee flexed	45
Hyperextension	15

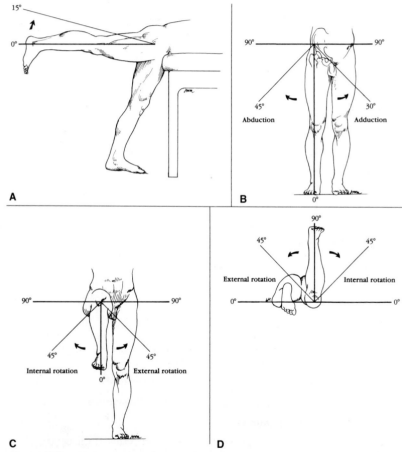

Figure 13–13. Passive range of motion of the hip. A. Extension. B. Lateral motion. C. Rotation in flexion. D. Rotation in extension (prone).

D. **Evaluate the hip for range of motion and tenderness and crepitation when client demonstrates range of motion** (Table 13–6).

1. **Instructions to client.** Be prepared to maneuver hip as instructed.

2. **Technique.**

    a. **To test rotation with extension.** With leg fully extended, roll leg laterally and medially. Flex hip and knee to 90 degrees and move knee laterally and medially to test rotation with flexion.

    b. **To test abduction.** Start with leg in extension. Grasp ankle and move leg laterally as far as possible.

    c. **To test adduction.** Start with leg in extension and neutral position. Move leg medially across opposite leg.

    d. **To test flexion.** Move knee toward chest as far as possible.

    e. **To test hyperextension.** The client is turned to the prone position. Raise leg posteriorly by grasping ankle and raising leg. Repeat with the examiner's fingers placed deep in the inguinal area to assess crepitation.

3. **Note** tenderness, crepitation, and limitation of motion.

4. **Normal findings.** Smooth, full range of motion (Fig. 13–13); nontender; no crepitation; flexion of the hips in the geriatric client.

5. **Clinical alterations**

    a. Pain, crepitus, and limitation of movement from osteoarthritis.

    b. Tenderness on range of motion owing to rheumatoid arthritis and bursitis.

True leg length will vary for the same leg, depending on its position in the abduction-adduction plane. Both legs should be placed in the same relative position for measurement.

Apparent leg length (inequality in the presence of equal true leg length) is due to pelvic tilt.

Legg-Calvé-Perthes disease. Aseptic necrosis of the femoral head usually occurring in children.

Circumference is measured to assess quadricep atrophy. The measurement is generally made 4 inches (10 cm) proximal to the superior border of the patella.

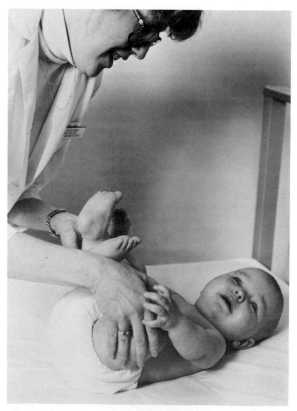

Figure 13–14. Assessment of hip dislocation in a 6-month-old infant.

E. **Compare leg length.**

   1. **Equipment.** Measuring tape.

   2. **Technique.** Measure distance from anterior superior iliac crest to medial malleolus for the true leg length.° Measure the distance from the umbilicus to the medial malleolus for the apparent leg length.° The tape should cross the knee on the medial sides.

   3. **Note** equality in length of the two legs.

   4. **Normal findings.** Leg lengths should be within one-half inch of each other.

   5. **Clinical alteration.** Shortening of one limb associated with *Legg-Calvé-Perthes disease* or dislocation of hip.

F. **Evaluate for muscle mass.**

   1. **Technique.** Measure the circumference° of the thighs making certain the measurement is made at symmetric levels above the knee.

   2. **Note** loss of muscle mass and difference in circumference between the legs.

   3. **Normal findings.** Measurements equal bilaterally; decreased muscle bulk in geriatric client.

   4. **Clinical alteration.** Atrophy associated with a diseased hip or compression of a nerve.

G. **Evaluate the hip for dislocation in infants.**

   1. **Technique.** Place infant in supine position. Fully flex hips and knees (Fig. 13–14). Abduct knees until lateral knees touch examining table.

   2. **Note** a click as the femoral head enters the acetabulum from a posterior position.

   3. **Normal findings.** No palpable or audible click.

   4. **Clinical alteration.** Congenitally acquired dislocation.

H. **Thoroughly examine the back and knee if client has hip pain.**

I. **Examine the abdomen and rectum if pain is present and the history is appropriate.**

J. **Common clinical alterations.** See **XVI.**

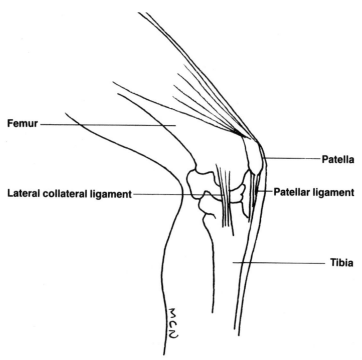

Figure 13–15. Right knee joint.

Evaluation of the knee should include questions about pain, instability, clicking, restricted movement, locking, swelling, deformity, and stiffness.

Genu varum. The knees deviate outward and the legs deviate toward midline, commonly referred to as bowleg.

Genu valgum. The knees deviate inward and the legs deviate away from midline, commonly referred to as knock knee.

Prepatellar bursitis (housemaid's knee). Localized swelling from chronic trauma to the knee.

By systematically palpating the knee, the major bursae of the knee will be palpated. In addition, the insertion of major ligaments will be palpated.

Osgood-Schlatter disease. Pain in the knee seen in overweight, adolescent boys.

If depressions of the knee are obliterated, the knee should be examined for effusion. Areas distal and proximal to the knee should be milked toward the patella. Light percussion on one side should demonstrate a fluid wave on the opposite side if fluid is present.

XI. **Evaluation of the knee.**° **Position** client so that he or she is standing.

A. Inspect the knee (Fig. 13–15).

1. **Technique.** Systematically inspect the knee anteriorly, posteriorly, medially, and laterally.

2. **Note** the alignment of the femur, tibia, and patella; soft tissue; thigh; color; level of popliteal creases; and muscles.

3. **Normal findings.** Bilaterally symmetric; without deformities; symmetric muscle mass smooth; hollowness adjacent to and above the patella. The knee should be straight when the sole of the foot contacts the ground. The levels of the patellae and the popliteal creases are equal. Flexion of the knees and loss of muscle bulk are seen in the geriatric client. ***Genu varum*** is seen in infants, ***genu valgum*** in children between 2 and 10 years of age.

4. **Clinical alterations**

   a. Genu varum in children more than 2 years of age.

   b. Genu valgum in adolescents and adults.

   c. Muscular atrophy.

   d. Swelling in the prepatellar area associated with ***prepatellar bursitis.***

   e. Fluid in the knee from blood, pus, or excess synovial fluid.

B. Palpate the knee.

1. **Instructions to client.** Describe any tenderness.

2. **Technique.** Systematically° palpate the patella, lateral and medial femoral condyles, tibial tuberosity, lateral and medial tibial condyles, and head of the fibula. The patellofemoral joint is examined by manually displacing the patella medially while the quadriceps are relaxed, and pressing laterally to the displaced patella. Palpate the area of the suprapatellar pouch on each side of the quadriceps and progress to the popliteal area and flexor tendons.

3. **Note** heat, swelling, obliteration of bony landmarks, bony or doughy enlargement, tenderness, atrophy, and hypertrophy.

4. **Normal findings.** Smooth; nontender.

5. **Clinical alterations**

   a. Tenderness and enlargement of the tibial tuberosity suggestive of ***Osgood-Schlatter disease.***

   b. Swelling on either side of the patella owing to synovial thickening or effusions.°

Table 13–7. Normal range of motion of the knee

Motion	Range (degrees)
Flexion	135
Extension	0
Hyperextension	10

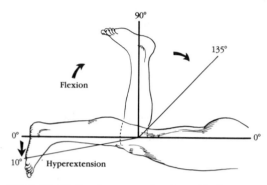

Figure 13–16. Passive range of motion of the knee.

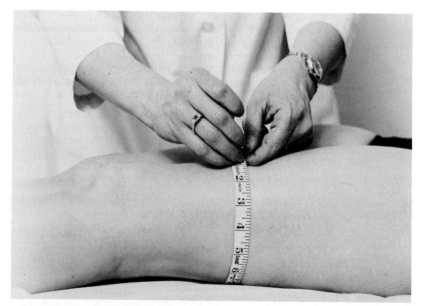

Figure 13–17. Measuring the circumference of the thigh to assess muscle mass.

    c. Doughy enlargement often from the hypertrophied joint of rheumatoid arthritis.

    d. Swelling and pain in the popliteal area associated with a popliteal abscess, semimembranous bursitis, Baker's cyst, or neuromyofibroma.

C. Evaluate the knee for range of motion and tenderness and crepitation when client demonstrates range of motion (Table 13–7).

    1. **Instructions to client.** Be prepared to maneuver knee as instructed.

    2. **Technique.** Palpate knee by cupping hand over anterior knee as client flexes knee and extends it.

    3. **Note** tenderness, crepitation, and limitation of motion.

    4. **Normal findings.** Full, smooth range of motion (Fig. 13–16); nontender; bilaterally equal; no crepitation.

    5. **Clinical alteration.** Tenderness and crepitation owing to degenerative joint disease, chondromalacia, or loose bodies in the joint.

D. Evaluate muscle mass.

    1. **Equipment.** Tape measure.

    2. **Technique.** Measure the circumference of the thigh 4 inches (10 cm) above the superior border of the patella (Fig. 13–17).

    3. **Note** atrophy and symmetry.

    4. **Normal findings.** Symmetric decreased muscle bulk in the geriatric client.

    5. **Clinical alteration.** Atrophy associated with a diseased knee or a compression of a nerve.

Knee injuries are common. The mechanism of injury should be obtained.

Injury to the cruciate ligaments commonly occurs with dashboard injuries.

Varus deformity. A deformity in which the knees are deviated outward and the legs are deviated toward midline. In the maneuver described in **H.1**, the lateral joint space widens.

Valgus deformity. A deformity in which the knees are deviated inward and the legs are deviated away from midline. In the maneuver described in **H.1**, the medial joint space widens.

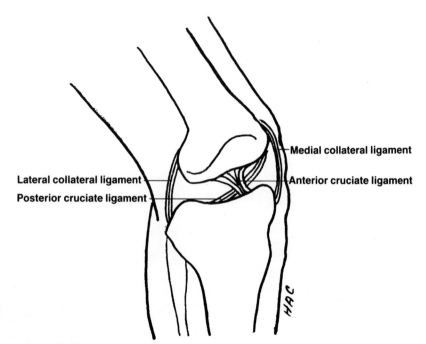

Figure 13–18. Anatomic location of the ligaments of the knee (patella and bursa not shown in order to expose ligaments).

E. **Thoroughly examine the hip, back, foot, and ankle if client has knee pain.**°

F. **Common clinical alterations.** See **XVI.**

Note: If anomalies are suspected, proceed to G and H. If not, proceed to I.

G. **Assess stability of the cruciate ligaments** (Fig. 13–18).°

1. **Technique.** Flex the knee to 90 degrees. Stabilize the foot. Attempt to displace the proximal end of the tibia forward by grasping the leg posteriorly and pulling forward. Attempt to displace the proximal end of the tibia backward by applying pressure posteriorly against the tibia.

2. **Note** deformity and pain.

3. **Normal findings.** No displacement.

4. **Clinical alterations**

    a. *Varus deformity.*

    b. *Valgus deformity.*

    c. Tenderness in the affected ligament and decreased lateral mobility from rupture of a collateral ligament.

    d. Locking and crepitus associated with a loose body in the joint.

    e. Instability of the knee joint owing to rupture of a cruciate ligament.

H. **Assess stability of the collateral ligaments.** (See Fig. 13–18.)

1. **Technique.** Flex the knee to 30 degrees. Stabilize the femur by placing hand on the medial aspect of the thigh. Apply slight pressure laterally. With the other hand grasp ankle and apply adduction force. Repeat the procedure by placing hand on the lateral aspect of the thigh. Grasp the ankle and apply abduction force.

2. **Note** deformity and pain.

3. **Normal findings.** Absence of pain and no deformity.

4. **Clinical alterations.** See **G.4.**

I. **Common clinical alterations.** See **XVI.**

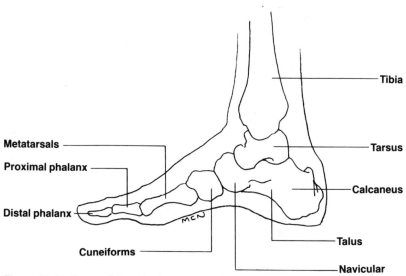

Figure 13–19. Bones of the right foot.

Medial malleolus. The distal tibia.

Lateral malleolus. The distal fibula.

XII. Examination of the ankle (Fig. 13–19). **Position** client so that he or she is supine.

A. **Inspect the ankle.**

   1. **Technique.** Systematically inspect the ankle posteriorly, anteriorly, medially, and laterally.

   2. **Note** color, swelling, edema, bony deformities, and nodules.

   3. **Normal findings.** Symmetric; no swelling or deformity.

   4. **Clinical alteration.** Swelling from arthritis, sprain, or fracture.

B. **Palpate the ankle.**

   1. **Instructions to client.** Describe any tenderness.

   2. **Technique.** Palpate the ankle anteriorly, posteriorly, medially, and laterally. Identify the ***medial*** and ***lateral malleoli,*** the calcaneus, and the Achilles tendon. Palpate the navicular bone, which is 1⅓ inches (3.5 cm) anterior to the medial malleolus. Palpate the talar neck anterior to the lateral malleolus with the foot plantar flexed and inverted. Palpate the cuneiforms on the dorsal surface articulating with the metatarsals. Palpate the cuboid immediately proximal to the fifth metatarsal.

   3. **Note** heat, swelling, edema, bony enlargement, deformities, obliteration of bony landmarks, tenderness, bogginess, and nodules.

   4. **Normal findings.** Smooth; nontender; bilaterally symmetric.

   5. **Clinical alterations**

      a. Nodules on the Achilles tendon seen in rheumatoid arthritis.

      b. Swelling and tenderness owing to arthritis, sprain, or fracture.

The ankle joint and the tibiofibular joint allow for dorsiflexion and plantar flexion; the subtalar joint and the talocalcaneal allow for inversion and eversion.

Table 13–8. Range of motion of the ankle

Motion	Range (degree)
Inversion	35
Eversion	25

Rapid range of motion may be checked by having the client walk on the toes, on the heels, and with the foot inverted and everted.

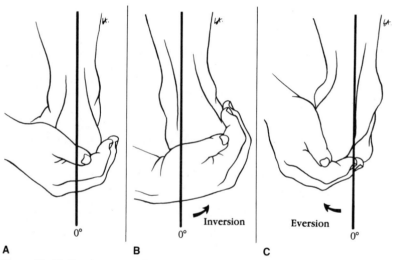

A   B   C

Figure 13–20. Passive range of motion of the ankle. A. Neutral. B. Inversion (left foot). C. Eversion (left foot).

An examination of the foot should include examination of the shoe. The shoe provides important information about the foot and ambulation. Wear should be more evident posterolaterally on the heel and under the foot medially. If the client is a jogger, his or her athletic shoes should also be examined.

Hammer toes. Hyperextension of the metatarsophalangeal joint and flexion of the proximal interphalangeal joint, often affecting the second toe.

Corn. Thickened skin caused by chronic pressure or irritation, usually found on the toes.

Callus. Thickened skin caused by chronic pressure, usually found on the sole.

Talipes. Pedal deformity.

C. **Evaluate the ankle for range of motion° and tenderness and crepitation when client demonstrates range of motion** (Table 13–8).

1. **Instructions to client.** Be prepared to maneuver ankle as directed.

2. **Technique.** Palpate ankle by cupping heel firmly in hand. With opposite hand, dorsiflex foot by drawing foot toward client's head and plantarflex by moving foot toward the ground. Invert ankle by turning foot inward and evert ankle by turning foot outward.

3. **Note** tenderness, crepitation, and limitation of motion.

4. **Normal findings.** Smooth, full range of motion (Fig. 13–20); no tenderness or crepitation.

5. **Clinical alterations**

   a. Pain only on inversion suggests chronic tenosynovitis or sprained ankle.

   b. Pain and limitation of range of motion from traumatic fracture.

   c. Instability owing to tears in ankle ligaments.

D. **Thoroughly examine the back, hip, and knee if ankle pain is present.**

E. **Common clinical alterations.** See **XVI.**

XIII. **Examination of the foot and toes** (see Fig. 13–19). **Position** client so that he or she is standing with shoes and socks removed.°

A. **Inspect the foot.**

1. **Technique.** Systematically inspect the foot and toes. Inspect alignment of the vertical axis of the heel with the calcaneus tendon.

2. **Note** posture and contact with the ground, the medial arch, and the alignment of the heel and foot.

3. **Normal findings.** Preservation of the arch, alignment of the heel with the tendon, and the foot pointing forward.

4. **Clinical alterations**

   a. *Hammer toes.*

   b. *Corn* or *callus.*

   c. *Talipes.*

   d. Decreased amounts of hair owing to peripheral vascular disease.

   e. Erythema and swelling of the metatarsophalangeal joint of the great toe suggestive of gout.

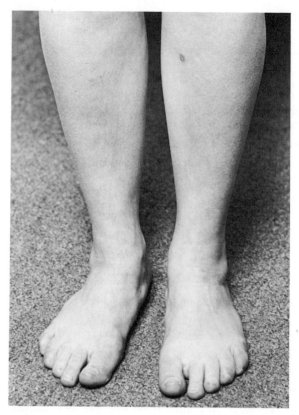

Figure 13–21. Inspection of the foot and leg.

Heads of the metatarsals. Commonly referred to as the ball of the foot.

Stress fractures or "marcher's fractures" are commonly seen in joggers.

B. **Inspect the foot and the leg.**

1. **Position.** The client sits with legs and feet hanging free.

2. **Technique.** The client then stands (Fig. 13–21). Systematically inspect the foot and posture.

3. **Note** the alignment of the patella with the first interdigital space, erythema, cyanosis, pallor, swelling, bony deformities, malalignment, callosities, warts, ulcers, varicosities, and lack of hair.

4. **Normal findings.** The patella aligns with first interdigital space. Foot should be straight and in slight plantar flexion. Toes should be straight, extended, and smooth. Adduction of the forefoot distal to the metatarsal-tarsal line is seen in children less than 2 years of age.

5. **Clinical alterations.** See **A.4.**

C. **Palpate the foot and toes.**

1. **Instructions to client.** Describe any tenderness.

2. **Technique.** Palpate along each metatarsal and each metatarsophalangeal joint. Compress the foot laterally between thumb and fingers at the level of the metatarsophalangeal joints. Compress each metatarsophalangeal joint by placing thumb on dorsal surface and fingers on plantar surface. Palpate the *heads of the metatarsals* on the plantar surface. Palpate the medial arch.

3. **Note** heat, swelling, tenderness, and bony deformities.

4. **Normal findings.** Smooth; nontender.

5. **Clinical alterations**

   a. Stress fractures° often in the second metatarsal.

   b. Pain suggestive of rheumatoid arthritis or bunion.

   c. Tender big toe associated with gout.

Table 13–9. Range of motion of the foot: dorsiflexion is 25 degrees and plantar flexion 45 degrees.

Joint	Flexion (degrees)	Extension (degrees)
First metatarsophalangeal	45	70–90
Metatarsophalangeal, of lesser toes	—	70–90
Proximal interphalangeal, of great toe	90	—
Interphalangeal of lesser toes	70–90	—

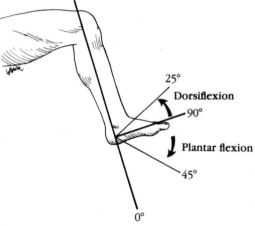

Figure 13–22. Passive range of motion of the ankle: dorsiflexion and plantar flexion.

D. **Evaluate the foot and toes for range of motion and tenderness and crepitation when client demonstrates range of motion.** (Table 13–9).

1. **Instructions to client.** Maneuver toes as asked.

2. **Technique.** Position foot such that the metatarsophalangeal joints are between the thumb and fingers. Flexion is accomplished by having the client curl the toes under; extension by having the client straighten the toes. The client should then fan the toes.

3. **Note** tenderness, crepitation, and limitation of motion.

4. **Normal findings.** Smooth, full range of motion (Fig. 13–22); bilaterally equal; nontender; no crepitation.

5. **Clinical alteration.** Pain on motion from arthritis or stress fracture.

E. **Thoroughly examine the back, hip, knee, and ankle if client has foot pain.**

F. **Common clinical alterations.** See **XVI.**

Observing ease of movement will give the examiner clues about any pain or limitations.

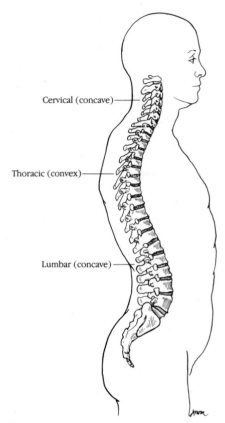

Figure 13–23. Normal spinal contours.

Scoliosis. Lateral curvature of the spine.

Lordosis. Accentuation of the normal posterior concavity.

Kyphosis. An exaggerated thoracic convexity, more common in women.

XIV. Examination of the back. Position client so that he or she is standing.

   A. **Observe the posture, gait, and ease of movement.**° **Observe the client while disrobing.**

   B. **Inspect the back.**

    1. **Technique.** Systematically inspect the back from the front, back, and sides. Having the client bend forward may accentuate abnormal curvatures.

    2. **Note** color; ecchymosis; alignment; cervical, thoracic, and lumbar curvatures (Fig. 13–23); symmetry in height of the shoulders; iliac crests; prominence of the scapulae; ribs and flanks; localized swellings; and scars.

    3. **Normal findings.** Spine is straight. Loss of height may occur as client ages. Kyphosis of aging may be present. Decreased thoracic convexity and increased lumbar concavity is seen in children.

    4. **Clinical alterations**

       a. *Scoliosis.*

       b. Flattened curvatures in the presence of muscle spasm.

       c. *Lordosis.*

       d. *Kyphosis.*

       e. Loss of height from thinning of the intervertebral discs and shortening or collapsed vertebral bodies.

   C. **Palpate the back.**

    1. **Instructions to client.** Describe any tenderness.

    2. **Technique.** Palpate the paravertebral muscles. Make long, gentle sweeping movements to assess subtle muscle spasm. Knead the paravertebral muscles between the fingers.

    3. **Note** heat, swelling, muscle spasm, deformities, tenderness, and asymmetry.

    4. **Normal findings.** Nontender; without spasm.

    5. **Clinical alterations**

       a. Tenderness from arthritis or herniated disk.

       b. Muscle atrophy owing to compression of motor nerves.

Table 13–10. Range of motion of the spine

Motion	Range (degrees)
Flexion	75–90
Extension	35
Lateral bending	30
Rotation	45

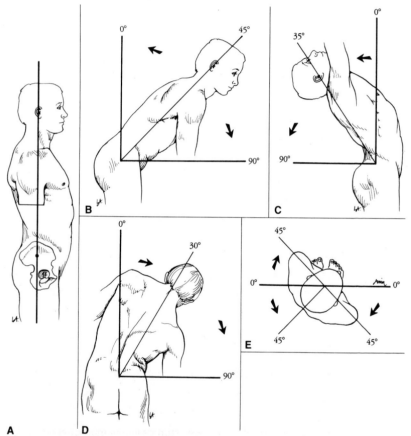

Figure 13–24. Passive range of motion of the lumbar spine. A. Normal. B. Flexion. C. Extension. D. Lateral bending. E. Rotation.

Low back pain is a common clinical entity with approximately 80 percent of the population experiencing this complaint at some time in their lives. It is generally self-limiting with remission of pain within 2 months in 90 percent of patients.

Spondylolisthesis. Forward slippage of L-5 onto S-1.

D. Evaluate the back for range of motion and for tenderness and crepitation when client demonstrates range of motion (Table 13–10).

1. **Instructions to client.** Be prepared to maneuver the body as directed.

2. **Technique**

   a. **Cervical spine.** See **V.**

   b. **Lumbar spine** (Fig. 13–24).

      (1) **To test flexion.** Have client bend forward from the waist as far as possible. Examiner's hand is positioned on the lumbar area as client moves forward. Alternate technique: Measure 4 inches (10 cm) up and 2 inches (5 cm) down from the level of the posterior superior iliac spines. Have client bend forward as much as possible. Measure distance previously marked. With flexion the distance should increase from 6 inches (15 cm) to 8 inches (20 cm) or greater.

      (2) **To test extension.** Have client return to the upright position. Stabilize client's hips by holding firmly and have client bend backward from the waist toward examiner.

      (3) **To test lateral bending.** Have client bend to each side as far as possible keeping both feet flat on the floor.

      (4) **To test rotation.** Stabilize the pelvis and have client twist the trunk from the waist.

3. **Note** limitation of motion, tenderness, and crepitation.

4. **Normal findings.** Smooth, full range of motion, nontender, no crepitations.

5. **Clinical alteration.**° Tenderness and decreased motion owing to ankylosing spondylitis, *spondylolisthesis,* herniated disc, or fracture of the vertebral body.

E. Percuss the spine.

1. **Position.** Client sits or stands with slight flexion.

2. **Equipment.** Rubber hammer.

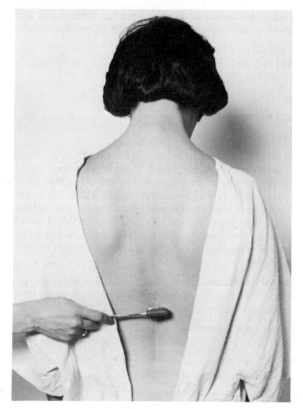

Figure 13–25. Percussion of the lumbar spine.

Radicular pain with straight leg raising would point to nerve root involvement.

The joints should be auscultated because fine crepitations may be auscultated in the absence of palpable crepitus.

3. **Technique.** Percuss each spinous process with a rubber hammer (Fig. 13–25).

4. **Note** tenderness.

5. **Clinical alteration.** Pain often indicative of disorder in the respective vertebra.

F. **Compare leg lengths.** See **X.E.**

Note: If pain is present, proceed to **G.** If not, proceed to **XV.**

G. **Assess sacroiliac joint.**

1. **Position.** The client is on his or her side.

2. **Technique.** Compress the sacroiliac joint by firmly pressing down on the pelvis.

3. **Alternate technique.** With client supine firmly rock pelvis against examining table.

4. **Note** tenderness.

5. **Normal findings.** No tenderness.

6. **Clinical alteration.** Tenderness from sacroiliac strain or sacroiliac arthritis.

H. **In the presence of pain, include the following:**

1. Examination of the hip.

2. Examination of the abdomen.

3. Examination of the rectum (in men more than 45 years of age).

4. Examination of the pelvis (if clinically indicated).

5. Straight leg raising. Particular attention should be made to the type and position of pain elicited with this maneuver.° The maneuver should be performed when client is both supine and sitting.

I. **Common clinical alterations.** See **XVI.**

XV. **Auscultate the joints.°**

A. **Instructions to client.** Maneuver joint through range of motion as directed previously.

B. **Equipment.** Stethoscope.

C. **Technique.** Place the diaphragm of the stethoscope over the joint to be auscultated as the client demonstrates range of motion.

D. **Note** fine crepitation.

E. **Normal findings.** None.

F. **Clinical alteration.** Crepitus from arthritis, osteoarthritis, or a loose body in the joint.

Notes

XVI. Common clinical alterations

   A. Erythema. Suggests bursitis, tendinitis, injury, rheumatoid arthritis, gouty arthritis, suppurative arthritis, and pseudogout (knee, wrist).

   B. Swelling. Suggests bursitis, tendinitis, dislocation, subluxation, fracture, tendon rupture or tear, soft tissue injury, ganglion, joint effusion, suppurative arthritis, rheumatoid arthritis, and gouty arthritis.

   C. Nodules suggest rheumatoid arthritis, osteoarthritis, gout, and repeated trauma.

   D. Tenderness. Suggests bursitis, tendinitis, dislocation, subluxation, fracture, tendon or ligament rupture or tear, soft tissue injury, nerve compression, rheumatoid arthritis, gouty arthritis, suppurative arthritis, neoplasms, and osteomyelitis.

   E. Limited range of motion (with pain, swelling, or both). Suggests dislocation, subluxation, fracture, tendon or ligament rupture or tear, rheumatoid arthritis, and osteoarthritis.

   F. Limited active range of motion with full passive range of motion. Suggests rotator cuff or other ligament or tendon ruptures or tears.

   G. Crepitation. Suggests arthritis, loose body, and fracture.

   H. Deformity. Suggests congenital deformity, dislocation, subluxation, fracture, rheumatoid arthritis, and osteoarthritis.

   I. Decreased muscle mass. Suggests immobilization, disuse, neuromuscular disorders, and aging.

   J. Paresthesias. Suggest carpal tunnel syndrome or other nerve involvement and gouty arthritis.

   K. Warmth. Suggests osteomyelitis, suppurative arthritis, gouty arthritis, rheumatoid arthritis, tendinitis, and bursitis.

   L. Contractures. Suggests disease, ischemia, and inflammatory processes.

XVII. Chart. Joints and surrounding tissues grossly symmetric, without erythema, swelling, and deformities; no tenderness, heat, palpable or audible crepitus, or joint extensions; range of motion full; joints stable.

Assessment of the Neurologic System

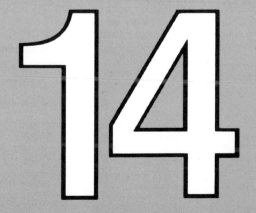

14

Functional divisions of the nervous system

1. The central nervous system (CNS) consists of the brain (for interpretation and direction) and the spinal cord (for reflex activity). It receives information sent from the environment through the peripheral and autonomic sensory pathways. It then processes and interprets the information according to prior learning and experience to initiate and direct a response, which is then sent out to the appropriate peripheral or autonomic motor pathway. There is no regeneration if parts of the CNS are destroyed.

2. The peripheral nervous system consists of the cranial nerves and the spinal nerves, which have branches that are distributed to various parts of the body for voluntary muscle action. It brings information to and from the CNS. Dysfunction of motor pathways will prevent effective use of the involved body part. If injury occurs, there is some recovery and regeneration. In selected circumstances use can be regained with the assistance of electrical devices.

3. The autonomic nervous system has two divisions, sympathetic and parasympathetic, with branch distribution to the body for smooth muscle and glandular action. Its fibers are responsible for the "automatic" functions of the body (e.g., secretions, heart rate, and digestive motions). Autonomic fibers travel in CNS and peripheral pathways so if those pathways are impaired, autonomic function will suffer. In selected circumstances, control of autonomic function can be assisted with medication.

Handedness. Handedness usually identifies hemisphere dominance. Ninety-nine percent of right-handed people are left-hemisphere dominated as are 60 percent of left-handed people.

Occupational status. People who use motor skills should be proficient in those skills. Sedentary persons may test within the normal range but may not demonstrate a high level of proficiency. Missed work time may indicate malingering. Frequent accidents may indicate a motor deficiency, seizure disorder, or sensory deficit (e.g., sight, hearing). The presence of illness may affect performance. Compatability of occupation to educational level indicates ability to perform. Exposure to heavy metals or toxic chemicals may be responsible for neurologic symptoms. Some neuromuscular symptoms can be caused by positional rigidity or repetitive motions required in some occupations.

I. Clinical considerations

A. The examiner should possess a conceptual understanding of the functional divisions of the nervous system° and a basic knowledge of nerve impulse conduction to correlate findings.

B. Examination of the nervous system includes assessment of cerebral function and sensorimotor function through inspection, palpation, and percussion.

C. It is helpful if the examiner demonstrates the maneuver the client is asked to perform.

D. Symmetry is essential to assess when examining the neurologic system.

E. When testing cranial nerves, do all eye tests and all mouth tests together to save time and avoid client fatigue. Itemize and record findings according to the particular nerve involved.

F. Advise the client that the intent of a sensorimotor examination is serious. Frank answers to questions and cooperation in performing requested activities are necessary.

G. Because all body functions are controlled by the nervous system, many aspects of sensorimotor function can be tested simultaneously during the routine health assessment as history is elicited and regions of the body are examined for abnormalities.

H. Maturational development should be correlated throughout the examination of the child.

II. Relevant history questions

A. *Handedness.*

B. *Occupational status.*

1. Use of motor skills versus sedentary.

2. Amount of time missed because of accident or illness.

3. Occupation compatible with educational achievement level.

4. Exposure to heavy metals or other toxic substances.

History of illness or injury. Family history is important as many conditions are hereditary. The following disorders may cause neurologic symptoms:

1. Diabetes mellitus is a major cause of sensory alterations.

2. The pain of herpes zoster can persist after rash has disappeared (postzoster syndrome).

3. Head injury can cause persistent residual neurologic deficits.

4. Limb injury may cause alterations in sensorimotor ability.

5. Late syphilis can affect cerebral and sensorimotor function, especially gait.

6. Seizure activity or postictal state may explain certain behavior changes.

7. Psychiatric disorders are sometimes treated by medications that may alter behavior or motor function.

8. Allergic reactions can explain or precipitate some symptoms or sensations.

9. Difficulty with motor coordination can be inherited.

Personal habits of alcohol, tobacco, and drug use often indicate the temperament of the client.

Use of leisure time may reflect neurologic capacity, degree of anxiety, or personal drive.

Complaints of altered sensation: The presence of pain may indicate obstruction or pressure. Loss of smell often follows a head injury. Loss of vision may indicate retinopathy or intracranial pressure. Loss of taste is often combined with loss of smell. Numbness and tingling indicate a neurosensory deficit.

Complaints of altered motor function indicate a probable neurosensory disorder, intracranial pressure, cranial nerve dysfunction, upper or motor neuron disease, or a muscular disorder.

C. *History of illness or injury* affecting motor ability or sensation in self or family.

1. Diabetes mellitus
2. Herpes zoster (shingles)
3. Head injury
4. Limb injury
5. Syphilis
6. Seizures
7. Psychiatric disorders
8. Allergies
9. Coordination disorder

D. **Personal habits.**°

1. Alcohol
2. Tobacco
3. Drug use (prescription or over-the-counter medication such as amphetamines, phenothiazines, neurotransmitters, barbiturates, narcotics, hypnotics, antibiotics, aspirin or other analgesics)

E. **Leisure time activity:**° active use of motor skills versus sedentary activities.

F. **Complaints of altered sensation.**°

1. Pain (site, description)
2. Smell (absence, exaggeration, hallucination)
3. Vision (blindness, diplopia, field deficit, hallucination)
4. Taste (loss, hallucination)
5. Numbness or tingling (site, description)

G. **Complaints of altered motor function.**°

1. Weakness (site, description)
2. Paralysis (site, description)
3. Balance (description)
4. Chewing difficulty (description)
5. Swallowing difficulty (description)
6. Muscle atrophy
7. Involuntary movement (site, description)
8. Difficulty with coordination (description)
9. Difficulty with facial expression

It is important to first assess mental function to correlate findings to the sensorimotor portion of the neurologic examination. If disorientation is severe, it may not be possible to continue testing mental status.

Orientation is usually lost first in the sphere of time, then place, and finally person.

Organic brain syndrome. Presenting symptoms of functional neurotic or psychotic syndromes caused by toxic or metabolic, inflammatory, or structural brain disorders.

Memory can be assessed within the context of the health history. Memory should be initially assessed because recall will affect responses given during the entire mental status examination.

Serial sevens require calculation rather than rote memory; it tests, however, only the client's ability to subtract.

   10. Difficulty speaking (lips, tongue, palate, hoarseness)

   11. Difficulty with sphincter control (bowel, bladder)

H. For all identified alterations, elicit the following:

   1. Character of onset (sudden, insidious)

   2. Associated circumstances (occupational, seasonal, time of day, related to specific activity, following a stressful event)

   3. Duration (occurred only once, existing since birth, recent, long term)

   4. Severity (interference with sleep or activities of daily life)

   5. Trends (persistent, intermittent, improving, worsening)

   6. Use of therapeutic modalities (prescribed or self; effectiveness)

   7. Associated signs and symptoms implicating possible nervous system disorder

III. Assessment of mental status. Position client so that he or she is seated in a comfortable chair (client should be dressed).

   A. Evaluate orientation.°

      1. Instructions to client. I will be asking you a series of questions; please answer as correctly as possible.

      2. Technique. Ask client his or her name, the date (including year), place, and day of the week.

      3. Note ability to respond correctly.

      4. Normal findings. Oriented in all three spheres of person, time, and place.° Orientation may be decreased in the geriatric client.

      5. Clinical alteration. Disorientation from **organic brain syndrome,** sensory deprivation, or a radical change in environment (i.e., hospitalization).

   B. Assess memory and ability to compute.°

      1. Instructions to client. I am going to give you verbally a series of numbers; repeat as many of them as you can remember. Next, repeatedly subtract seven, beginning at 100 (i.e., 100, 93, 86, and so forth).° Lastly, I will tell you three things that I want you to remember. Listen carefully and repeat them to yourself. I will ask you to repeat them at various times throughout the examination.

      2. Technique. Verbally give the client a random series of digits, one every second. Tell the client three unrelated words (i.e., orange, address, horse). Ask client to repeat them in 3 minutes, 10 minutes, and 30 minutes.

      3. Note client's ability to compute and recall.

Language function. The ability to receive and interpret information and to send appropriate messages. It should be assessed after memory because the client's ability to comprehend and express himself or herself will influence the rest of the examination. Impaired hearing will decrease client's response to the assessment of language function.

Aphasia. A language disturbance, often following a stroke, in which the client fails to understand language or makes errors using it.

Dysarthria. Imperfect articulation of speech owing to disturbances of muscular control that result from damage to the central or peripheral nervous system.

Proverb interpretation requires an intact fund of information plus the ability to apply it.

An example of an abstract response to proverb is, "It takes a long time if things are to be done well."

An example of a concrete response is, "You can't build a city over night" (literal interpretation.)

4. **Normal findings.** Client can repeat a digit span of 6 to 7 forward and 4 to 5 backward and subtract serial sevens. Client has no difficulty learning new material or recalling it later. Memory may be slightly decreased in the geriatric client.

5. **Clinical alterations**

   a. Impaired digit span and serial sevens associated with organic brain syndrome.

   b. Impaired ability to remember words owing to mental retardation, depression, dementia, anxiety, thiamine deficiency, chronic alcoholism (Korsakoff's syndrome), or head injury.

   c. Loss of remote memory during health interview because of dementia.

C. **Assess *language function*.**

   1. **Equipment.** Printed cards with separate matching pictures.

   2. **Instructions to client.** Match the word on this card to the picture it best describes. Point to an object I name (i.e., clock, pen).

   3. **Note** ability to interpret directions.

   4. **Normal findings.** Client able to match correctly words with pictures and to point to the correct objects. Smooth, flowing speech; clear expression of thoughts.

   5. **Clinical alterations**

      a. *Aphasia* from diffuse cortical damage or early stages of a progressive lesion.

      b. Slow speech owing to mental retardation or depression.

      c. Rapid, animated speech associated with mania.

      d. *Dysarthria* owing to demyelinating disease.

      e. Empty content speech associated with dementia or psychosis.

D. **Measure abstract reasoning ability.°**

   1. **Instructions to client.** I will quote a saying with which you may or may not be familiar; please explain in your own words what the saying means.

   2. **Technique.** Ask the client what is meant by the saying, "Rome wasn't built in a day."

   3. **Note** relevance of answer and degree of concreteness.

   4. **Normal findings.** Abstract or semiabstract response.°

   5. **Clinical alteration.** Concrete response° owing to schizophrenia, organic brain syndrome, or mental retardation.

Judgment can be assumed intact if the client is in touch with reality, has been managing his or her family and business affairs, and is in no financial or legal difficulty.

In evaluating the client's ability to make decisions regarding judgment, the examiner should give a situation appropriate to his or her educational and socioeconomic background.

All aspects of the client's appearance and behavior should be assessed throughout the entire examination.

Family and close friends may be helpful or not helpful (may be accustomed to behavior).

A client may demonstrate mild anxiety when being interviewed, particularly if he or she is fearful of being ill.

E. **Assess judgment.**°

1. **Instructions to client.** I am going to give you an imaginary situation. Please tell me what you would do.

2. **Technique.** Ask the client what he would do if he were driving down the street and saw the second story of an apartment building on fire.°

3. **Note** judgment in solving the situation.

4. **Normal findings.** Able to realistically make the proper decisions, thinking of the safety of others.

5. **Clinical alterations**

   a. Impaired judgment with mental retardation, organic brain syndrome, mania, or depression.

   b. Egocentric self-preservation or impulse indulgence owing to dementia, psychosis, or immaturity.

F. **Examine general appearance and behavior.**°

1. **Technique.** Observe client throughout the examination. Talk with family and close friends.°

2. **Note** general grooming, weight, gestures and affect; facial expression; psychomotor retardation or hyperactivity; disorganized behavior; and any peculiar movements.

3. **Normal findings.** Client relaxed and composed throughout interview;° willing to answer questions.

4. **Clinical alterations**

   a. Increased activity associated with mania.

   b. Saddened, depressed mood owing to depression.

   c. Elated or irritable owing to mania.

   d. Tense or hyperactive because of anxiety or phobic disorders.

   e. Poor grooming because of organic brain syndrome, depression, or schizophrenia.

   f. Fastidiousness because of an obsessive compulsive disorder.

   g. Dull affect associated with organic brain syndrome.

   h. Flat affect in the schizophrenic client.

Cranial nerves. Twelve pairs of nerves (each side of the body receives one-half of each pair) that originate in the brain and exit toward the periphery. Classified as sensory, motor, or mixed according to function, cranial nerves supply branches to the head and neck areas of the body.

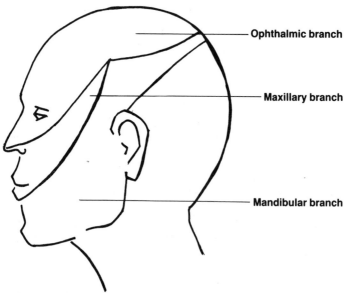

Figure 14–1. Cutaneous innervation of the head.

Trigeminal nerve (fifth cranial nerve). Provides mixed motor and sensory function through three branches: (1) ophthalmic, (2) maxillary, and (3) mandibular. The trigeminal nerve provides motor function to muscles of mastication and sensory function (touch, pain, and temperature) to face and mucosa of eyes, nose, and mouth.

Amyotrophic lateral sclerosis (ALS; sometimes called Lou Gerhig's disease). A disorder caused by progressive loss of motor cells, which can cause either upper or lower motor neuron signs (or both) depending on whether cortex, brainstem, cranial nerves, corticospinal (pyramidal) tract, or anterior roots are involved. Pull is to the strong side with weakness and atrophy on weak side so affected side will deviate.

Tic. Repetitive, rhythmic movement of a muscle or a group of muscles (e.g., grimacing, winking, head or shoulder movements).

Fasciculations. Small, rapid wormlike contractions of muscles, visible through the skin, representing a spontaneous discharge of a number of fibers innervated by a single nerve filament. Fasciculations are seen in lower motor neuron dysfunction.

IV. Testing of *cranial nerve* function

A. **Elicit alterations in sensation (smell, vision, taste, hearing); motion (weakness, paralysis, abnormal movements); and autonomic function (gag, cough) in the head, neck, and shoulders.**

1. **Equipment.** Tissues, cotton-tipped applicators, aromatic solutions in small bottles (lemon, peppermint, and clove oils; coffee); penlight; Snellen chart; cardboard eye shield; ophthalmoscope; pin (having sharp and dull ends); tongue blades; tuning fork; small containers with clean solutions of glucose, saline, and vinegar; gauze sponge; and paper cup.

2. **Position.** Client seated comfortably in a chair.

3. **Instructions to client.** I will be testing sensation and movement in and around your face. I will need your cooperation in looking at lights, opening your mouth, closing your eyes, and moving your head and shoulders. It will not be painful.

B. **Assess the function of the optic nerve (second cranial nerve).** See Chapter 6, **III.L.** and **IV.A–B.**

C. **Assess the function of the oculomotor (third cranial nerve), trochlear (fourth cranial nerve), and abducens nerve (sixth cranial nerve) and ophthalmic branch of the trigeminal nerve (fifth cranial nerve).** See Chapter 6, **IV.E.**

D. **Assess the function of the *trigeminal nerve* (fifth cranial nerve)** (Fig. 14–1).

1. **Motor component**

a. **Instructions to client.** Be prepared to make several facial motions when asked to do so.

b. **Technique.** Observe relaxed face for symmetry of jaws. Cradle client's cheeks by placing palms of both hands alongside the jaws with fingers against temples. Palpate masseter and temporal muscles as client clamps and relaxes jaws.

c. **Note** strength of masseter, temporal, and pterygoid muscles and deviation of jaw.

d. **Normal findings.** Symmetric jaws with face at rest; ability to open and close jaws with equal strength; absence of involuntary movements.

e. **Clinical alterations**

(1) Inability to close jaw owing to bilateral weakness seen with lower motor neuron disease (***amyotrophic lateral sclerosis***) or neuromuscular disorders (myesthenia gravis).

(2) Lateral deviation of jaw from trauma or brain lesions.

(3) *Tic.*

(4) *Fasciculations.*

Temperature sensation. Ability to distinguish between hot and cold. Temperature, pain, and touch sensations are conducted through shared pathways. If damage occurs, it is usually deep touch that is lost first; therefore, temperature sensation can be assumed to be intact if the client can feel a pin prick.

Tic douloureux. Trigeminal neuralgia.

Herpes zoster (shingles). An acute and painful inflammatory disease of the cranial or posterior nerve root ganglia and peripheral nerves. It is caused by the varicella virus.

Facial nerve (seventh cranial nerve). Provides motor function to muscles of facial expression, sensory function for taste on anterior two-thirds of tongue, and parasympathetic fibers for salivary and lacrimal glands and mucosa.

2. Sensory component

a. Equipment. Wisp of cotton or cotton-tipped applicator. Hot and cold water in capped test tubes.

b. Instructions to client. Close your eyes. Each time you feel something, say "Yes," and then tell me where I touched you and whether the sensation was sharp, dull, or feathery.

c. Technique. Using a cotton wisp, touch several random points in each branch distribution on both sides of face including lips, inside mouth, and nose. Repeat the procedure, this time with a pin prick alternating with dull side of pin in random fashion. Test to **temperature sensation** only if doubtful about pain or touch sensations.

d. Note response to stimulation by light touch and pain in all three branches of nerve distribution.

e. Normal findings. Response appropriate to stimulation applied.

f. Clinical alterations

(1) Anesthesia in one or all areas of branch distribution caused by brain lesions following injury or surgery.

(2) Hypersensitivity or report of facial pain seen with **tic douloureux** or after **herpes zoster.**

E. Assess the motor function of the *facial nerve* (seventh cranial nerve).

1. Instructions to client. Please perform the following maneuvers when asked to do so.

a. Raise your eyebrows as high as you can.

b. Close your eyes tightly, do not let me pull them open.

c. Frown and wrinkle your nose.

d. Show your teeth in a snarl.

e. Smile (spontaneously).

f. Puff out your cheeks.

g. Whistle.

2. Technique. Observe client's face in repose and when performing actions described in **1.** Tap the bone just anterior to the ear above the parotid gland on one side. Repeat on other side.

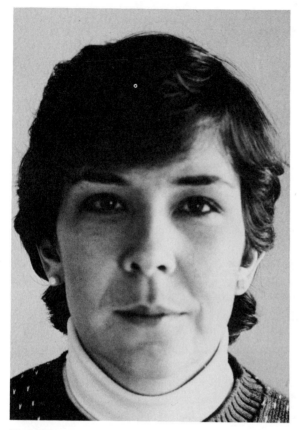

Figure 14–2. Assess the face in repose for symmetry.

Spasm. A sudden involuntary contraction of a muscle or group of muscles.

Tremor. Involuntary trembling or quivering, described as fine if the vibrations are rapid and coarse if the vibrations are slow. It should be noted whether tremor occurs at rest (resting tremor) or during voluntary activity (intention tremor).

Bell's palsy. A lower motor neuron disorder of the facial nerve resulting in unilateral facial paralysis. In most cases the cause is unknown.

Chvostek's sign. A spasm of the facial muscles elicited by tapping the facial nerve.

Some examiners also test the client's ability to detect bitter with quinine.

If client has difficulty maintaining protrusion, assist by holding tip of tongue with a gauze sponge.

3. **Note** facial symmetry (Fig. 14–2); presence of tearing, drooling, or **spasm;** facility of facial movements; and **tremor** of eyelids.

4. **Normal findings.** Many people have a slightly asymmetric face but weakness and difficulty with facial expressions are not normal.

5. **Clinical alterations**

   a. Drooping or weakness at rest or with facial expressions.

   b. Flattening of nasolabial fold on either side.

   c. Tearing or drooling seen with **Bell's palsy,** stroke, and some muscular dystrophies.

   d. **Chvostek's sign** because of hypocalcemia.

F. **Assess the function of the sensory component of the facial nerve (seventh cranial nerve) and the sensory component of the glossopharyngeal nerve (twelfth cranial nerve) for taste.**

1. **Instructions to client.** I am going to check your ability to taste. There are three important things you need to do.

   a. Keep your tongue protruded.

   b. If you taste something, raise your right hand.

   c. Look at this paper and point to the substance you tasted.

2. **Technique.** Hand client a piece of paper on which are written the words *salty, sweet,* and *sour.*° Dip cotton-tipped applicators into solutions of saline, glucose, and vinegar (acetic acid). Do not allow client to view labels. Place wet saline applicator on anterior two-thirds section of one side of tongue. Wait for response.° Repeat using glucose on opposite side of tongue. Place wet vinegar applicator on posterior one-third section of one side of tongue. Repeat randomly until both sides of tongue have been tested with all solutions.

3. **Note** client's ability to taste solution and to recognize it appropriately on both sides of tongue.

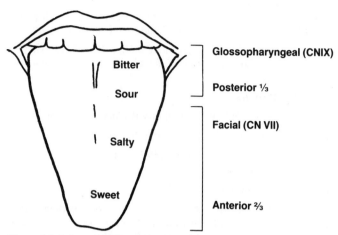

Figure 14–3. Location of taste buds on the tongue.

Hyperacusis. An exceptionally acute sense of hearing; everything seems loud. Branches of the facial nerve innervate the stapedius muscle and those of the glossopharyngeal nerve innervate the tympanic membrane and eustacian tube. As they exit from the brainstem, both these nerves are located near the acoustic nerve, and hearing is affected if lesions are present.

4. **Normal findings.** Sense of taste intact bilaterally to salty, sweet, and sour substances (Fig. 14–3).

5. **Clinical alteration.** Inability to taste is rare; may result from skull trauma; significant if ***hyperacusis*** is also present.

G. **Assess the function of the olfactory nerve (first cranial nerve).** See Chapter 4, **III.D.**

H. **Assess the function of the vagus nerve (tenth cranial nerve) and the motor component of the glossopharyngeal nerve.** See Chapter 4,**IV.M.**

I. **Assess the function of the acoustic nerve (eighth cranial nerve).** See Chapter 5,**III.G–J** and 14,**V.B.**

J. **Assess the function of the accessory nerve (ninth cranial nerve).** See Chapter 3,**VI.C.**

K. **Assess the motor component of the hypoglossal nerve (twelfth cranial nerve).** See Chapter 4,**IV.E.**

Shoes should be removed because they may alter posture or gait.

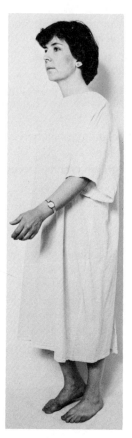

Figure 14–4. Observation of gait with shoes removed.

Chorea. Rapid, sudden, jerky, involuntary movements that occur at irregular, unpredictable intervals (unlike tics), without rhythm or repetition. The movements stop during sleep.

Spastic hemiparesis. Muscular weakness or paralysis affecting one side of the body. Arm on affected side is held tightly flexed against body. There is stiffness of the affected leg with plantar flexion of the foot causing a semicircular leg swing and dragging of the toe as the person steps forward.

Spastic diplegia (Little's disease). Bilateral paralysis. The knees are held together and steps are abnormally short and effortful (scissors gait).

Waddling. Wide-based stance and the trunk is displaced backwards from lumbar lordosis. The client appears to waddle and wiggle in attempt to remain upright.

V. Assessment of motor function

A. Identify alterations of gait.

1. **Instructions to client.** Remove shoes.° Please perform the following activities as directed. The geriatric client may need to be assisted when performing these maneuvers.

   a. Walk back and forth across the room (or up and down hallway) using your normal stride (Fig. 14–4).

   b. Hop on one foot, then the other.

   c. Walk in a straight line touching the heel of your leading foot against the toe of your following foot (tandem walking).

2. **Note** posture, balance, swing of arms in relation to step, coordination of body movements, fashion in which foot makes floor contact, and presence of involuntary movements in trunk and extremities.

3. **Normal findings.** Client able to maintain erect posture; smooth, free swing of opposite arm with each step; foot makes contact with floor in a heel-toe fashion; may need visual assistance to perform tandem walking; able to hop on each foot; no involuntary movements. Performance may be altered in the elderly because of other physical disability (e.g., arthritis).

4. **Clinical alterations**

   a. Inability to stand owing to weak leg muscles.

   b. *Chorea* seen with lower motor neuron disorders.

   c. *Spastic hemiparesis* owing to unilateral upper motor neuron disorder in the cerebral cortex (i.e., stroke).

   d. *Spastic diplegia* because of disease involving upper motor neurons (i.e., cerebral palsy and multiple sclerosis).

   e. *Waddling* commonly seen in myopathies.

Steppage gait. The client lifts the affected foot high, then brings it down with a slap owing to foot drop.

Hypotonia (tabetic). Diminished tone of the muscles. The stance is broad based and the knee joints are unstable. The legs are lifted high and slapped down firmly and the client watches each step.

Ataxia. Irregularity in muscular action, which results in a wide-based stance and unsteady gait. Client staggers and has difficulty turning.

Parkinsonism. Hypokinesia, tremor, and muscular rigidity. Posture appears stooped; there is flexion of the hips, elbows, and knees. General mobility is decreased owing to rigidity. Steps are short and shuffling. Client has difficulty initiating steps and then stopping (once begun).

Hysteria. A psychogenic disorder marked by emotional instability and various sensory and motor disturbances. Varied and bizarre in character and does not consistently resemble an abnormal gait produced by organic nervous system disease.

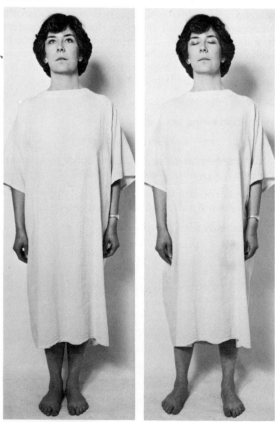

A   **B**

Figure 14–5. Testing for Romberg's sign. Note the ability of the client to stand erect with eyes open (A) and closed (B).

f. *Steppage gait* commonly seen with lower motor neuron disorders (spinal cord segments and peroneal neuropathy).

g. *Hypotonia* commonly seen in disorders of the dorsal columns of the spinal cord (if it is due to tabes dorsalis, the client will have a positive serologic test for syphilis.)

h. *Ataxia* often from cerebellar disorders, peripheral neuropathy, or toxicity from alcohol, barbiturates, or heavy metal.

i. *Parkinsonism* associated with disorders of the basal ganglia.

j. *Hysteria* seen in the client who has a secondary gain motivation (i.e., attention, disability pay).

B. **Test for Romberg's sign** (Fig. 14–5).

1. **Instructions to client.** Put both feet together and stand with eyes opened, then close eyes.

2. **Note** client's ability to maintain an upright posture with feet together when eyes are opened and then closed.

3. **Normal findings.** Client able to stand erect with minimal swaying.

4. **Clinical alterations**

   a. Inability to maintain upright position only occurring with eyes closed often associated with a loss of position sense (dorsal column), a vestibular disorder, or injury to the acoustic nerve.

   b. Inability to maintain upright position occurring with eyes open often associated with a cerebellar deficit.

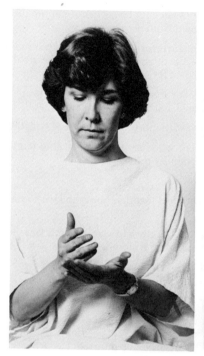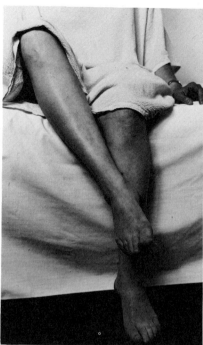

Figure 14–6. Testing motor coordination of the upper extremities (left) and the lower extremities (right).

Dyssynergia. Loss of coordination in performing motor acts; movement is jerky rather than smooth.

Athetosis. A slow writhing and twisting motion seen with cerebral palsy. Movement stops during sleep.

Myoclonus. A sudden, rapid, unpredictable involuntary movement. It is associated with some seizure disorders but sometimes occurs in normal individuals while they are falling asleep. A hiccup is a myoclonic movement of the diaphragm.

Dysdiadochokinesia. Difficulty in performing rapid alternating movements.

Dysmetria. Inability to judge distance and to stop movement at a chosen spot; the client will over or under reach. It is also termed *past pointing*. Because it can be due to either a visual or coordination problem, it is important to correlate findings.

C. **Test coordination.**

   1. **Position.** Client seated with both feet on the floor. Examiner standing 18 inches (46 cm) in front of and facing the client.

   2. **Instructions to client.** Perform the following activities when asked:

     a. **Upper extremities**

       (1) Pat the palms of both hands against your thighs, go faster and faster.

       (2) Pat one palm at a time, faster and faster. Alternate right, left, right, left (Fig. 14–6).

       (3) Pat with both hands, first palms down, then palms up, faster and faster.

       (4) Touch your thumb on opposition against each finger, go back and forth in rapid succession.

       (5) Close eyes, extend arms, alternately touch nose with index fingers. Do the same with your other hand.

     b. **Lower extremities**

       (1) Tap both feet on the floor, go faster and faster.

       (2) Tap one foot, then the other; go faster and faster. Alternate.

       (3) Pick up your right foot and run your heel down your left shin from knee to ankle (see Fig. 14–6).

       (4) Switch sides and do the same.

   3. **Note** smoothness and accuracy of movement, confusion and involuntary movement.

   4. **Normal findings.** Client able to perform all requested movements accurately and smoothly in both upper and lower extremities without confusion or involuntary movement. Movements may be somewhat slower in the elderly.

   5. **Clinical alterations.** Difficulty performing repetitive movement of upper or lower extremities or both because of the following:

     a. *Dyssynergia*

     b. Tremors

     c. *Athetosis*

     d. *Myoclonus*

     e. *Dysdiadochokinesia*

     f. Fasciculation

     g. *Dysmetria*

Table 14–1. Innervation of the muscles of the upper extremities

Upper Limb Muscles	Nerve	C2	C3	C4	C5	C6	C7	C8	T1
Sternocleidomastoid; trapezius	Spinal accessory	X	X	X					
Diaphragm	Phrenic		X	X	X				
Deltoid	Axillary				X				
Supraspinatus	Suprascapular				X				
Infraspinatus	Inferior scapular				X	X			
Teres minor	Axillary				X	X			
Subscapularis; teres major	Subscapular				X	X			
Serratus anterior	Long thoracic				X	X	X		
Rhomboideus	Dorsal scapular				X				
Clavicular pectoralis major	Anterior thoracic				X	X	X		
Biceps; brachialis	Musculocutaneous				X	X			
Brachioradialis	Radial				X	X			
Latissimus dorsi	Thoracodorsal					X	X	X	
Sternopectoralis major	Anterior thoracic					X	X	X	X
Flexor carpi radialis; pronator teres	Median					X			
Extensor carpi radialis, longus & brevis; extensor digitorum communis; extensor indicis proprius; extensor carpi ulnaris; extensor pollicis, longus & brevis; abductor pollicis longus; triceps	Radial					X	X	X	
Flexor digitorum sublimis	Median						X	X	X
Flexor digitorum profundis	Volar interosseous; ulnar						X	X	
Flexor carpi ulnaris	Ulnar						X		
Pronator quadratus	Volar interosseous							X	X
Dorsal interosseous; volar interosseous	Ulnar							X	
Lumbricals; flexor pollicis brevis	Median; ulnar							X	X
Adductor pollicis brevis; opponens	Ulnar							X	X
Biceps tendon reflex	Musculocutaneous				X	X			
Extensor pollicis tendon reflex	Radial						X		
Triceps tendon reflex	Radial						X	X	

Tone. The sensation of resistance felt by the examiner during passive manipulation of the client's relaxed joint.

VI. Testing of range of motion of all muscles and joints. See Chapter 13.

VII. Assessment of *tone* and strength of proximal and distal muscles of the upper extremities (Table 14–1). **Instruct** client that strength of various muscles will be tested. Client will be asked to flex and hyperextend various muscles and to maintain flexion against resistance.

Most people are right-handed and the side of the handedness is normally stronger. In testing the upper extremities, it is a good idea to consider this and to criss-cross hands (as in a handshake) or to approach from the rear.

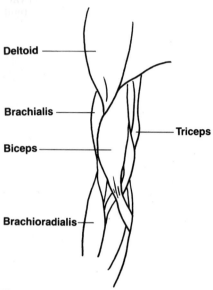

Figure 14–7. Anatomic location of muscles of the upper extremity.

A. Assess the deltoid muscle (Fig. 14–7).

1. **Position.** Stand behind the client with dominant hand° grasping client's dominant distal humerus just above the elbow.

2. **Technique.** Passively flex and extend client's relaxed arm several times. Apply pressure and request that the client maintain arm in abduction against resistance.

B. Assess the triceps muscle (Fig. 14–7).

1. **Position.** Face client and assume an arm wrestling position by grasping client's wrist with your hand.

2. **Technique.** Passively flex and extend client's relaxed supinated arm several times. Provide resistance against flexed arms and request that the client push examiner away by extending his or her arm.

C. Assess the biceps muscle (see Fig. 14–7).

1. **Position.** See **B.1.**

2. **Instructions to client.** Make a muscle.

3. **Technique.** Grasp wrist and pull down as client attempts to maintain flexion of arm.

D. Assess the brachioradial muscle (see Fig. 14–7).

1. **Position.** Continue holding client's wrist but position arm halfway between pronation and supination.

2. **Technique.** Repeat passive flexion and extension. Apply counterpressure and repeat active flexion and extension.

E. Assess finger flexors (grip).

1. **Instructions to client.** Grip my fingers as hard as you can. Do not let my fingers go as I attempt to release them.

2. **Technique.** Place index and middle fingers in the client's palm. Laterally pull away from client's grip.

F. Assess wrist flexors.

1. **Instructions to client.** Make a fist with your hand and bend your wrist down (as if knocking) so your knuckles point to the floor. Hold your hand down, do not let me pull it up.

2. **Technique.** Grasp client's hand and pull up as client attempts to maintain flexion against resistance.

G. Assess wrist extensors.

1. **Instructions to client.** Keep your hand fisted but this time make your knuckles point to the ceiling and do not let me pull your hand down.

2. **Technique.** Grasp client's fisted hand and pull down as client attempts to maintain hyperextension against resistance.

Table 14–2. Scale for evaluating and recording muscle strength (power)

Grade	Description
0	No contraction
1	Flicker or trace of contraction
2	Active movement, with gravity eliminated (cannot maintain against gravity)
3	Active movement against gravity but no resistance
4	Active movement against gravity with slight resistance
5	Normal active movement against gravity with good resistance

Rigidity. Stiffness and resistance to passive movement. There are two types:

1. Cogwheel: the resistance is subject to a series of rapid fluctuations owing to a superimposed effect of a tremor, causing alternating contraction and relaxation of the muscles being stretched.

2. Lead-pipe: the resistance is uniform with no fluctuation.

Clonus. A sustained series of involuntary contractions and relaxations of a muscle that occur in rapid succession. Its presence indicates spasticity.

H. Assess finger extensors.

   1. Position. Client seated with pronated arm resting on table and fingers over the edge.

   2. Instructions to client. Hold your fingers straight out and keep them there; do not let me bend them.

   3. Technique. Prevent wrist motion by placing two fingers on client's extended hand just distal to the wrist joint. With your other hand, extend two fingers and push them down laterally against resistance.

I. Switch to nondominant side and repeat all tests. Compare muscle strength.

J. Note bulk, power, and tone in proximal and distal muscles in all extremities and presence of tenderness on palpation. Use a scale of 0 to 5 (Table 14–2) to grade the strength of each muscle (or muscle group). Note the presence of an involuntary movement. Identify whether it is the proximal or distal muscles that are involved and look for correlations with other findings.

K. Normal findings. No muscle wasting; a grade of 5 in all muscles tested; no tenderness; no rebound phenomenon; no involuntary movement.

L. Clinical alterations

   1. Atrophy, hypotonia, or fasciculation seen in lower motor disorders.

   2. *Rigidity* seen in basal ganglia disorders (Parkinsonism).

   3. Spasticity or *clonus* seen in upper motor neuron disorders.

Table 14–3. Innervation of the muscles of the lower extremities

Lower Limb Muscles	Nerve	L1	L2	L3	L4	L5	S1	S2	S4	S5
Hip flexion	Iliopsoas; sartorius; rectus femoris; tensor fasciae latae	Lumbar plexus; femoral; superior gluteal; obturator	X	X	X	X				
Hip adduction	Adductor major; adductor brevis; adductor longus	Obturator		X	X	X				
Knee extension	Quadratus femoris	Femoral			X	X				
Hip abduction	Gluteus medias; gluteus minimus; tensor fascia femoris	Superior gluteal				X	X	X		
Foot inversion & dorsiflexion	Tibialis anterior	Peroneal				X	X			
Toe extension	Extensor digitorum, longus & brevis	Peroneal				X	X	X		
Great toe extension	Extensor hallucis, longus & brevis	Peroneal					X	X		
Foot eversion	Peroneus, longus & brevis	Peroneal					X	X		
Foot inversion & plantar flexion	Tibialis posterior	Tibial					X	X		
Toe flexion	Flexor digitorum, longus & brevis	Tibial					X	X		
Great toe flexion	Flexor hallucis longus	Tibial					X	X	X	
Hip extension	Gluteus maximus	Inferior gluteal					X	X	X	
Knee flexion	Biceps femoris; semimembranous; semitendinosis	Peroneal; tibial					X	X	X	
Foot plantar flexion	Gastrocnemius; soleus	Tibial						X	X	
	Cremasteric reflex	Genital-femoral	X							
	Patellar tendon reflex	Femoral			X	X				
	Achilles tendon reflex	Tibial						X	X	
	Anal reflex	Pudendal								X	

VIII. Eliciting of tone and strength of proximal and distal muscles of the lower extremities (Table 14–3). **Position** client so that he or she is lying supine and relaxed on examining table. Examiner is on right.

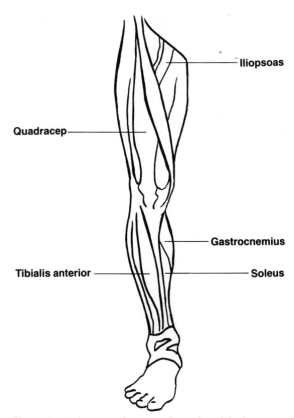

Figure 14–8. Anatomic location of muscles of the lower extremity.

A. Assess iliopsoas muscle (Fig. 14–8).

1. **Instructions to client.** Bend your leg when asked to do so; do not let me push it down.

2. **Technique.** Face client's feet. Place your left hand on client's right thigh. Place your right hand on client's heel and passively flex and extend client's leg and hip several times. With leg and hip in flexed position, push down with left hand as client attempts to maintain flexion against resistance.

B. Assess quadriceps muscle (see Fig. 14–8).

1. **Instructions to client.** Continue to keep your leg bent. Straighten your leg when asked to do so.

2. **Technique.** With client's leg still flexed at hip and knee, place your right hand on client's skin near the ankle. Push with hand as client attempts to extend leg against resistance.

C. Assess hamstring muscles (see Fig. 14–8).

1. **Position.** Client lying prone with feet over edge of the table.

2. **Instructions to client.** Bend your knee up. Do not let me pull it down.

3. **Technique.** Stand at the foot of table and grasp client's posterior ankle. Passively flex and extend client's leg at the knee several times. With client's leg flexed at the knee, pull on client's posterior ankle as client attempts to keep knee flexed against resistance.

D. Assess gastrocnemius muscle (see Fig. 14–8).

1. **Position.** Client lying supine with legs extended.

2. **Instructions to client.** Push my hand away when asked to do so.

3. **Technique.** Stand to one side, place palm on ball of client's foot, fingers toward client's heel. Push as client attempts to plantar flex foot against resistance.

E. Assess toe flexor muscle.

1. **Instructions to client.** Curl your toes down and push me away when asked to do so.

2. **Technique.** Place fingers on plantar aspect of client's extended toes. Provide resistance as client attempts to flex toes.

F. Assess soleus muscle (see Fig. 14–8).

1. **Instructions to client.** Bend your knee and push your foot against my hand.

2. **Technique.** Keep palm on plantar surface of client's foot. Request client to flex knee. Place other hand on client's thigh to stabilize leg. Provide resistance against foot as client attempts plantar flexion.

Reflexes	**Reflex Arc Level**
Brachioradial	Cervical 5, 6
Biceps	Cervical 5, 6
Triceps	Cervical 6, 7, 8
Patellar	Lumbar 2, 3, 4
Achilles	Sacral 1, 2

G. **Assess anterior tibial muscle** (see Fig. 14–8).

   1. **Instructions to client.** Pull your foot toward your head; do not let me push it down.

   2. **Technique.** Place hand on dorsal aspect of client's foot as it rests in anatomic position. Provide resistance as client attempts to dorsiflex foot.

H. **Assess toe extensors.**

   1. **Instructions to client.** Do not let me pull your toes down. Lift your leg in the air and trace a figure eight with your big toe when asked to do so.

   2. **Technique.** Place fingers on dorsal aspect of client's toes. Stabilize foot by placing other hand across client's ankle. Provide resistance as client attempts to keep toes extended.

I. **Switch to nondominant side and repeat all tests. Compare muscle strength.**

J. **Note.** See **VII.J.**

K. **Normal findings.** See **VII.K.**

L. **Clinical alterations.** See **VII.L.**

IX. **Testing of deep tendon and superficial reflexes.**

   A. **Elicit deep tendon reflexes (DTRs).°**

      1. **Equipment.** Reflex hammer.

      2. **Position.** Client seated on side of examining table.

      3. **Instructions to client.** I will be tapping you to test your reflexes. Please keep your joints relaxed. It will not hurt.

Reinforcement technique. A method of distracting a tense client. The conventional method is to ask client to pull one hand against the other with flexed fingers interlocking in a monkey grip (Jendrassik's maneuver) for lower extremity testing. If the tendon jerks of the upper extremity are being tested, the client is instructed to make a fist with the other hand.

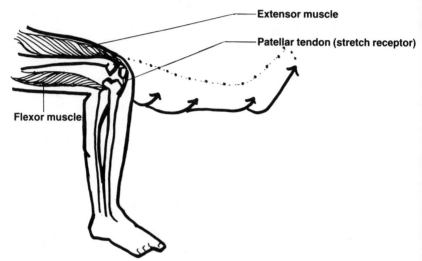

Figure 14–9. Stretch reflex of the patellar tendon.

For Achilles response, ask client to kneel on a chair with feet dangling off the edge, then tap the tendon.

Table 14–4. Scale for evaluating and recording tendon jerk responses

Grade	Description
0	No response
1	Low normal, slightly diminished response
2	Normal response
3	More brisk than normal; may indicate anxiety
4	Hyperactive with clonus

A normal response indicates that the reflex arc is intact at the spinal cord level on both afferent and efferent sides. A small percentage of persons normally have diminished or absent DTRs, especially elderly clients or those with arterial vascular problems.

Superficial reflexes. Receptors are located in the skin rather than the muscle tendons.

4. **Technique.** Using a reflex hammer, provide a brisk tap on the following muscle tendons (if unable to elicit a response for all upper extremities and patellar response, use *reinforcement technique*):

   a. **Brachioradial.** With client's arm resting in a position halfway between supination and pronation, tap the tendon just above the bony prominence of the wrist on the radial side.

   b. **Biceps.** Place your thumb on client's biceps tendon and with client's arm flexed, tap your thumb.

   c. **Triceps.** With client's arm in abduction and forearm hanging freely, tap on the tendon just above the elbow.

   d. **Patellar.** With client's leg flexed at the knee and the thigh stabilized by examiner's hand, tap the tendon below the kneecap (Fig. 14–9).

   e. **Achilles.** With client's foot slightly dorsiflexed and stabilized by examiner's hand, tap the tendon.°

5. **Repeat** on opposite side.

6. **Note** briskness of response and whether reinforcement technique was necessary to elicit a response. Use a scale of 0 to 4 (Table 14–4) to grade tendon jerk responses.

7. **Normal findings.**° Grade of 2 + for all DTRs with appropriate response to tap as follows:

   a. **Brachioradial.** Forearm, fingers, and hand should flex and supinate.

   b. **Biceps.** Arm should flex.

   c. **Triceps.** Arm should extend.

   d. **Patellar.** Leg should extend ("knee jerk").

   e. **Achilles.** Foot should plantar flex ("ankle jerk").

8. **Clinical alterations**

   a. Increased response, when correlated with hypertonia, suggests upper motor neuron disorders.

   b. Decreased response, when correlated with muscle wasting or hypotonia, suggests the flacidity seen with lower motor neuron disorders.

B. Elicit *superficial reflexes.*

   1. **Equipment.** Tongue blade or reflex hammer.

   2. **Position.** Client lying supine and relaxed.

   3. **Instructions to client.** I will be stroking your feet and abdomen with this tongue blade. Please stay relaxed. It will not hurt.

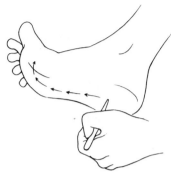

Figure 14–10. Technique of eliciting the Babinski reflex. The sole is stroked firmly along the path indicated.

Babinski reflex. Dorsiflexion of the big toe when the sole of the foot is stimulated. Its presence indicates suppressed cortical control and is a pathologic response in a person more than 2 years of age. It is a normal response of the immature nervous system in infancy.

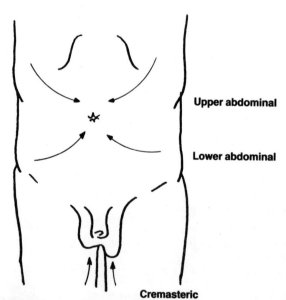

Figure 14–11. Direction of stroke when testing abdominal and cremasteric reflexes.

4. **Elicit plantar response.**

   a. **Technique.** Stabilize leg by placing one hand above client's ankle. Using tongue blade, lightly but firmly stroke the lateral aspect of client's sole, starting at the heel then moving toward the big toe. Repeat on the other foot (Fig. 14–10).

   b. **Note** response of toes as lateral aspect of sole is stroked and presence of *Babinski reflex.*

   c. **Normal findings.** Toes should flex.

   d. **Clinical alterations**

      (1) Decreased cortical control.

      (2) Upper motor neuron or pyramidal tract disease.

      (3) Amyotrophic lateral sclerosis.

5. **Elicit superficial abdominal reflexes** (Fig. 14–11).

   a. **Position.** Abdomen exposed.

   b. **Technique.** Briskly and lightly stroke tongue blade across one side of upper abdomen from lower outer rib cage toward umbilicus. Repeat on the other side. Stroke on a diagonal across lower abdomen from iliac fossa toward umbilicus. Repeat on the other side.

   c. **Note** position change of umbilicus toward side stoked.

   d. **Normal findings.** Umbilicus moves toward the source of stimulation. If the client is obese, multiparous, elderly, or recovering from recent abdominal operation, the response may be normally diminished.

   e. **Clinical alterations**

      (1) Diminished or absent response seen with peripheral neuropathies and spinal cord or nerve compression.

      (2) Unusually brisk responses seen in cerebral palsy.

6. **Test cremasteric reflex (in male client)** (see Fig. 14–11).

   a. **Position.** Genitalia and thighs exposed.

   b. **Technique.** Stroke the medial aspect of client's anterior thigh. Repeat on opposite side.

   c. **Note** position change of scrotum in response.

   d. **Normal findings.** Elevation of scrotum in response.

   e. **Clinical alterations**

      (1) Response diminished or absent with corticospinal tract lesions.

      (2) Brisk responses are found in children.

Testing sensation is difficult because of subjectivity. To conduct a proficient and reliable sensory assessment, the examiner must practice to attain dexterity and avoid cueing.

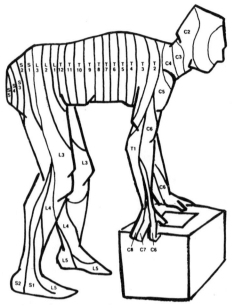

Figure 14–12. Segmental arrangement of dermatones representing nerve distribution entering and exiting the spinal cord from, and back to, the periphery at each of the 31 cord segments.

Compare with dermatome chart, map areas with alterations using a skin-marking pencil and proceed with testing of temperature sensation looking for patterns of alteration.

It is unnecessary to test temperature sense if response to pain is intact.

Alterations found should validate pain sense findings.

Alterations may represent lesions of dorsal column or spinothalamic tracts.

X. Assessment of sensory function: identifying alterations of sensation in trunk and extremities.° Necessary pieces of **equipment** are pin with sharp point and dull head; cotton wisp; tuning fork; small objects (various coins, key, button); a dermatome chart (Fig. 14–12); skin-marking pencil; two test tubes with stoppers. **Instruct** client that his or her ability to feel will be tested. Say, "Please keep your eyes closed. Each time you feel something, say 'Yes,' then tell me where I touched you and whether the sensation was sharp, dull, buzzing, feathery, hot, or cold."

A. Test pain sense.

   1. **Technique.** Using a pin, randomly touch client with sharp and dull side. Start in distal areas and move proximally. Repeat several times, varying touch locations. Persist until hands, forearms, upper arms, trunk, feet, lower legs, and thighs have been touched (do perineal and perianal areas if history reveals a sphincter problem).

   2. **Note** client's perception of sharpness and dullness in all areas tested. Correlate with sensory testing of trigeminal nerve. Compare corresponding areas on each side of the body, compare distal and proximal areas on the same side.

   3. **Normal findings.** Appropriate perception with no alterations indicates intact peripheral nerves and spinothalamic tract.

   4. **Clinical alterations**°

      a. Anesthesia, hypoesthesia, hyperesthesia.

      b. Peripheral neuropathy if in distal areas only, spinothalamic tract involvement if higher.

B. Test temperature sense.°

   1. **Technique.** Fill one test tube with cold water and the other with hot water.

   2. **Note** whether areas of alteration correspond with deficits of pain sensation.

   3. **Normal findings.** Client able to distinguish hot from cold.

   4. **Clinical alteration.** Loss of temperature sense, either hot or cold (more commonly hot) or both.°

C. Test light touch sensation.

   1. **Technique.** Using a cotton wisp, proceed with same technique as for testing pain sense.

   2. **Note** consistency of response in comparison to pain sense. Compare side to side for touch sensation.

   3. **Normal findings.** In all areas tested, light touch sense intact.

   4. **Clinical alteration.** Light touch sense may be diminished or lost earlier than pain sense in peripheral neuropathies.°

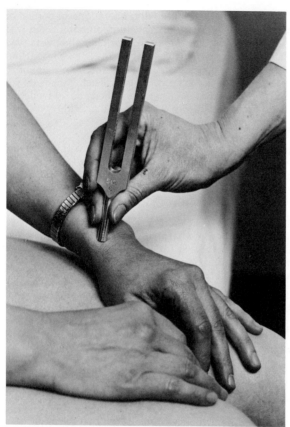

Figure 14–13. Testing vibration sense. Note how examiner places the tuning fork over the bony area of the wrist.

D. Test vibration sense.

1. **Instructions to client.** In addition to telling me the type of sensation you feel, tell me when the sensation stops.

2. **Technique.** Using a tuning fork, randomly touch bony areas of client's arms, legs, and trunk (Fig. 14–13). Periodically, and in random fashion, stop the vibration by pinching the prongs of the tuning fork. Persist until both wrists, elbows, shoulders, rib cage, ankles, shins, knees, and hips have been tested. Move distal to proximal.

3. **Note** any differences from side to side or distal to proximal; mark patterns of alteration with skin pencil.

4. **Normal findings.** Appropriate perception with no alterations indicates intact peripheral nerves and dorsal column tracts.

5. **Clinical alterations**

    a. Peripheral neuropathy.

    b. Lesions of dorsal columns.

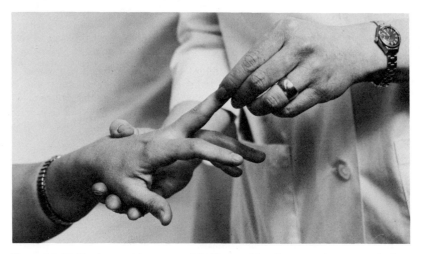

Figure 14–14. Testing position sense of the fingers. Note how examiner grasps both sides of the finger to avoid giving clues by pressure.

Validate results with findings on coordination tests.

Stereognosis. The ability to recognize objects on the basis of touch. It is a gross measure of sensory cortical function.

A small change purse containing pennies, dimes, nickels, quarters, paper clips, a key, and a button assists the efficiency of the examiner.

Aphasia. A disturbance of symbolic language, often following a stroke, in which the client either fails to understand language (sensory) or makes errors in using it (motor).

Two-point discrimination. Two simultaneous pin pricks are used to establish how far apart two pricks are perceived as two and not one.

Extinction phenomenon. Two corresponding body areas (right and left sides) are simultaneously pricked. A person should normally feel in both places. An impairment of the sensory cortex may cause the client to say that only one side has been pricked (extinction or denial on one side).

E. Test position sense (Fig. 14–14).

   1. **Instructions to client.** Please tell me whether I move your finger or toe up or down.

   2. **Technique.** Grasp the lateral aspect of client's digit (big toe, thumb, or any finger) and change its position from dorsiflexion to plantar flexion randomly, several times (return briefly to the neutral position before each change). Persist until one digit on all four limbs has been tested.

   3. **Note** accuracy and consistency of response; presence of any uncertainty or confusion.

   4. **Normal findings.** Able to perceive and identify directional change with accuracy.

   5. **Clinical alteration.** Slowness, hesitancy, or inability in reporting position change,° owing to posterior column disease.

F. Test tactile discrimination (*stereognosis*).

   1. **Instructions to client.** Please tell me the name of the object that I place in your hand.

   2. **Technique.** Place a key or a coin in client's hand. Test other side using a different object.°

   3. **Note** accuracy of response in naming objects and presence of hesitancy, confusion, or need to be prompted.

   4. **Normal findings.** Client must be able to correctly name the objects (dime, quarter, key, etc.) placed in both hands.

      a. A description of the objects ("to open a door," "money," etc.) is not an accurate response and may indicate *aphasia.*

      b. Astereognosis, which indicates a sensory problem requiring specific testing for *two-point discrimination* and *extinction phenomenon.*

      c. A cortical deficit (aphasia) requiring specific cerebral testing.

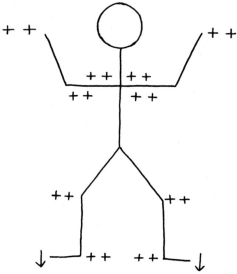

Figure 14–15. Chart of deep tendon reflexes and Babinski response.

XI. Chart. Cranial nerves grossly intact; smooth coordinated movements and gait; negative Romberg; motor strength 5+ bilaterally; deep tendon reflexes 2+ bilaterally; Babinski absent (Fig. 14–15); sensation intact to light touch and pain; abdominal reflexes present.

Index